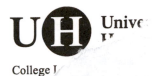
Unive
College I

911: Responding for Life

Case Studies in Emergency Care

911: Responding for Life

Case Studies in Emergency Care

Jim Whittle, BS
Coordinator of Paramedic and Fire Fighting Programs
Algonquin College
Ottawa, Ontario

Edited by
Bill Metcalf
Division Chief/EMS/Special Services
North Lake Tahoe Fire Protection District
Incline Village, Nevada

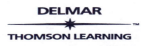

DELMAR

™

THOMSON LEARNING

Australia Canada Mexico Singapore Spain United Kingdom United States

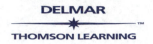

911: Responding for Life
by Jim Whittle, BS

Health Care Publishing Director:
William Brottmiller

Editorial Assistant:
Jill Korznat

Marketing Coordinator:
Penelope Cartwright

Executive Editor:
Cathy L. Esperti

Executive Marketing Manager:
Dawn F. Gerrain

Production Editor:
Mary Colleen Liburdi

Acquisitions Editor:
Marie M. Linvill

Marketing Channel Manager:
Tara Carter

Cover Design:
William Finnerty

Library of Congress
Cataloging-in-Publication Data
Whittle, Jim
911: Responding for Life

NOTICE TO THE READER

CONTENTS

This book is dedicated to all emergency medical technicians and paramedics who have shared their professional experiences and expertise by precepting students on ambulance field placements. The dedication and commitment demonstrated by EMTs who have taken students under their wing and provided guidance and the opportunity to learn in a positive and constructive environment ensures the continuity of what it means to be a professional in this field.

INTRODUCTION

The purpose of the case study format is to:

(A) Provide the reader with up-to-date knowledge by combining medical pathologies with actual case histories. The goal is to help the reader recognize important relationships between theory and practice.

(B) Test the reader's knowledge base and reasoning ability through critical thinking and a problem-solving approach. This will allow the reader to apply concepts and principles in new situations.

Case studies are beneficial not only for the relationship established between theory and practice, but, more important, for the critical thinking and problem-solving approach they take. This approach enables the emergency medical technician (EMT) or paramedic to be confronted by several problems simultaneously and to identify priorities in both assessment and management.

Instead of overwhelming the health-care provider with the complexity of a situation, a critical thinking and problem-solving approach allows him or her to identify each component of the situation separately and to list these individual problems in order of priority. These can be distinguished as either actual or anticipated problems. Actual problems are those that require immediate intervention, while anticipated problems are those that do not yet exist but may require intervention in the future.

When reading and working through the cases contained in this book, it is important to approach them critically from a problem-solving base. There are several ways to do this:

1. Trial-and-error in problem solving—occurs without forethought or perception of relationships, but simply by means of chance and the process of elimination.
2. Scientific method of problem solving—uses deductive reasoning. It
   a) defines the problem
   b) collects data
   c) formulates an hypothesis
   d) tests hypothesis
   e) formulates conclusions

For obvious reasons, the trial-and-error method would be extremely costly in terms of patient welfare. The scientific method of problem solving can also be costly in terms of time and efficiency.

In order to determine which approach works best in medicine it is important to remember that the dynamics involved in providing emergency medical care are not based on the theoretical categorization of patients into units such as cardiac, respiratory, or neuro. We need to step outside the classroom and recognize that patients present themselves with signs and symptoms, and it is from these "complaints" that the puzzle can start being assembled. What is needed is a complaint-based approach to determine the "field diagnosis" and subsequent patient management. Critical thinking in this complaint-based problem-solving approach is the best method of providing optimum patient care.

3. Critical thinking in problem solving
   a) recognizes problem potential
   b) gathers and assesses information
   c) defines problem(s)
   d) projects potential outcomes
   e) selects a management plan
   f) implements plan of action
   g) evaluates plan and outcome

   The key to effective critical thinking and problem solving lies in the first step. Too frequently we rush over this part of the process, believing that we know (based on first impressions) what the problem is, only to learn later that we were working with a false premise. While gathering and assessing data, emergency responders are wise to keep an open mind about their definition of the problem, so that it can be validated or changed as needed. They gain insight when they evaluate their problem-recognition skills and the management outcome for future reference. For this reason the final step in the process, which includes debriefing each call and finding out the definitive diagnosis when possible, becomes essential in ensuring an ongoing standard of quality care. Over time, the combination of expertise and experience will enable the EMT to progress through the problem-management process with greater speed and finesse.

   A final note on what I think is an essential digression from the strictly clinical discussion just taken place. It is critical not to forget the human element of the equation, which most will say, comes down to treating all patients no matter what their circumstance with dignity and respect. This is a code of conduct to which all EMTs should subscribe. The human element, however, also keeps in mind that most EMTs are in this field because we have caring and compassionate natures. Knowing that many of the calls will ingrain themselves in our minds, it can leave us prone to "burn-out." We need to acknowledge that it is important to allow room for normal emotional responses.

   When a new recruit asked a veteran how he was able to get used to the trauma of a recent call, that of caring for the shattered body of a young child, the veteran's answer was simple and understated: "you hope you never do!"

CASE STUDY 1

The night sky was clear, allowing the full moon to shine down on the mostly deserted streets. It was Halloween and the little groups of ghosts and goblins had for the most part completed their rounds of trick-or-treating. The ambulance crew had sound educational backgrounds in the medical sciences, not the supernatural sciences, yet if asked whether they believed that a full moon made a difference in the number and nature of calls they were likely to see that night, they would both have stated without hesitation that it did. Experience had taught them to be prepared for the unexpected on a night like this. The call that came their way, however, was not atypical.

A call from a Mr. John Stark had been prioritized urgent but not life threatening. The responding crew pulled up in front of a townhouse at approximately nine in the evening. A young woman in her twenties opened the door and directed the EMTs to the living room, where a young man was lying on the couch. He stated that his name was John and seemed distressed at the arrival of the EMTs, saying that his girlfriend had insisted he call. The non-attending EMT walked across the room and turned off the rather loud sitcom on the television set, then began to gather information from the young woman.

The attending paramedic observed that John did not look well: he was pale and grimacing with obvious discomfort. He was alert and coherent, and identified his main complaint as diffuse abdominal pain which had been developing over the past few days. He said that the pain would come and go but had basically been without relief despite the dozen Tylenols that he had taken over the past two days.

John thought he might have a bad case of the flu, since he had been feeling sick for the last week and a half with a headache, fever, and fatigue. Currently, he complained of additional nausea, and aching in the joints. In addition, an unexplained rash was causing a fair bit of itching. He admitted to being a smoker but said that he had not touched a cigarette since the day before, which was unusual since he always smoked, even when he had a cold.

John stated that he was twenty-eight years old and had been very healthy until now, playing both softball and basketball once a week. He had been employed at a computer firm for the past four years. He had no history of trauma, no major illnesses in the past, and he was not on any medication other than the self-prescribed Tylenol.

Focusing attention on the chief complaint (abdominal pain), John denied noticing any dysuria or hematuria, although he said his urine was dark in color, whereas his stools were greyish. He denied being a heavy drinker and stated that he did not do drugs. After conferring with the young woman, John revealed that he had eaten only once today, a bland meal of toast and soup, and he lost weight over the past few weeks having very little appetite. Neither relief nor additional pain had followed his meager meal, just increased nausea, which gave way to vomiting shortly thereafter.

With John's consent, the paramedic conducted a physical exam and noted no pulsating masses, discoloration, guarding, rigidity, or ascites. There was, however, tenderness on palpation of the right upper quadrant (RUQ). Assessment of vital signs provided the following information: pulse 96 regular and strong; respirations 22 regular with normal tidal volume; blood pressure 122/78; pupils equal and reactive to both direct and consensual light reflex; skin condition somewhat pale yet warm to touch; and a definite yellowish color to the sclera of the eyes. The ECG revealed a normal sinus rhythm without ectopy.

At this point, the paramedic ruled out abdominal trauma and suspected that the pain may be hepatic in origin. The patient was placed on supplemental oxygen and an IV was established with normal saline. John was placed in the position of comfort and transported to the hospital for further evaluation. Since his pain was not severe, the paramedic decided against initiating the pain management protocol.

Multiple-Choice Questions

1. Cirrhosis leading to hepatic failure often describes an etiology that includes:
1. chronic alcoholism
2. pancreatitis
3. hepatitis
4. cholecystitis

   a) 1, 3, 4
   b) 1, 2, 3
   c) 2, 3, 4
   d) 1, 2, 4
   e) all of the above

2. Which of the following non-prescription medications would most adversely affect the liver if taken in toxic amounts?

1. aspirin
2. Tylenol
3. acetaminophen
4. salicylate

   a) 1, 2
   b) 1, 3
   c) 1, 4
   d) 2, 3
   e) 2, 4

3. Which of the following statements concerning hepatitis A are true?

1. It often leads to chronic hepatitis.
2. It is transmitted through the oral-fecal route.
3. It is sometimes called infectious hepatitis.
4. It is the most debilitating form of hepatitis.

   a) 1, 3
   b) 2, 4
   c) 2, 3
   d) 1, 2, 4
   e) 1, 3, 4

4. Which of the following statements concerning hepatitis B are true?

1. It can be transmitted by contact with human secretions and feces.
2. It is sometimes called serum hepatitis.
3. Patients are most often asymptomatic.
4. This disease may be sexually transmitted.

   a) 2, 4
   b) 3, 4
   c) 1, 3, 4
   d) 1, 2, 3
   e) 1, 2, 4

5. Which of the following statements concerning hepatitis C are true?

1. formerly called post-transfusion non -A, non-B hepatitis
2. rarely progresses to chronic hepatitis
3. No vaccine is available.
4. Transmission includes IV drug use.

   a) 1, 2
   b) 2, 3
   c) 1, 3, 4
   d) 2, 3, 4
   e) 1, 2, 4

6. Which of the following statements are correct?
1. Hepatitis D can be contracted when the patient already has hepatitis B.
2. Hepatitis D may lead to chronic hepatitis and death.
3. Hepatitis E can be prevented with the vaccine for hepatitis B.
4. Hepatitis E does not result in chronic hepatitis.

    a) 1, 3
    b) 2, 4
    c) 1, 2, 3
    d) 1, 2, 4
    e) all of the above

7. Signs and symptoms commonly associated with hepatitis include:
1. bradycardia
2. fatigue
3. light-colored stools
4. light-colored urine
5. jaundice

    a) 1, 2, 3
    b) 2, 3, 5
    c) 1, 3, 4
    d) 2, 4, 5
    e) 1, 4, 5

8. Signs and symptoms commonly associated with hepatitis include:
1. nausea
2. abdominal pain
3. hyperventilation
4. fever
5. hypertension

    a) 1, 3, 5
    b) 2, 4, 5
    c) 3, 4, 5
    d) 1, 2, 3
    e) 1, 2, 4

9. Signs and symptoms commonly associated with hepatitis include:
1. dilated pupils
2. anorexia
3. pitting edema
4. hepatomegaly
5. arthralgia

    a) 1, 2, 4
    b) 1, 3, 5

c) 2, 3, 5
d) 2, 4, 5
e) 1, 3, 4

10. Which of the following statements concerning incubation and communicability are true?
1. Communicability for hepatitis A precedes the onset of symptoms.
2. Communicability for hepatitis B precedes the onset of symptoms.
3. Incubation for hepatitis A approximates 6 to 26 weeks.
4. Incubation for hepatitis B approximates 2 to 6 weeks.

a) 1, 2
b) 3, 4
c) 1, 3, 4
d) 2, 3, 4
e) all of the above

11. Which of the following statements concerning prognosis are true?
1. Hepatitis A is often fatal and the majority of those infected will become carriers.
2. Hepatitis B is rarely fatal and the majority of those infected will not become carriers.
3. Chronic hepatitis B is associated with liver cancer.
4. Lifelong immunity is provided with hepatitis A.

a) 1, 2
b) 1, 3
c) 3, 4
d) 1, 2, 4
e) 2, 3, 4

12. Preventive measures for hepatitis include which of the following?
1. vaccination for A, B, and C
2. washing hands after removing gloves
3. never contacting a patient with hepatitis
4. wearing a face mask at all times

a) 2
b) 1, 3
c) 1, 2
d) 1, 2, 4
e) 2, 3, 4

Debriefing

Body substance isolation (BSI) is the standard when dealing with any patient no matter what the etiology. The use of disposable gloves, worn at the outset, should be routine with all patients, as should be hand washing after each call. Remember as well that all linen should be discarded at the end of the call, according to protocol, to prevent indirect contamination.

In this particular case, the immediate danger of shock can be ruled out with a non-tachycardic pulse and a pulse pressure (difference between diastolic and systolic) of 44 mmHg. Very little is provided in terms of past history; indeed, other than smoking, John has been in relatively good health throughout his adult life. The chief complaint is essentially abdominal pain, which is not a helpful indicator of the cause. The best insight into the nature of John's problem comes from the assessment of signs and symptoms.

The absence of hematuria or melena helps point away from internal bleeding. Tenderness to palpation of the right upper quadrant (RUQ) with moderate hepatomegaly may indicate inflammation of the liver. The yellowish tinge to the sclera of John's eyes could be an early sign of jaundice giving further evidence of a possible liver ailment. Jaundice is the result of rising levels of bilirubin in the blood plasma. Failure of the liver cells first to take up and conjugate this orange bile pigment, and secondly to excrete it, is often part of the pathology of hepatitis.

In the field, it is very difficult to differentiate among all the possible illnesses. A chief complaint of abdominal pain makes differentiation all the more difficult. However, the paramedic is not expected to arrive at a definitive diagnosis. Nonetheless, taking complete and relevant histories, as well as thoroughly assessing all patients, will help to anticipate potential problems en route and provide for a continuity of care by providing essential information to the hospital staff.

The three clues discussed in this case scenario (tenderness in the RUQ, hepatomegaly, and jaundice) are the most distinguishing signs. Many of John's signs and symptoms could easily point in different directions; therefore, in order to problem-solve, it is important to find those features that distinguish this ailment from others. Indeed, most cursory examinations could easily conclude that John was simply suffering from a bad case of the flu.

Viral hepatitis is a fairly common systemic disease, which usually resolves without complications. In most patients hepatic cells eventually regenerate with little or no residual damage. Old age and serious underlying disorders will make complications more likely. Prognosis is poor, however, in those few who develop fulminant hepatitis characterized by hepatic encephalopathy.

Follow-Up

The crew (while wearing gloves) assisted John to the stretcher, which was placed semi-sitting for his comfort, with a basin in case of vomiting. He was placed on supplemental oxygen and an IV was started with normal saline. He was kept warm and taken to the hospital without incident.

Hospital diagnosis revealed hepatitis B in the early icteric phase. It was later discovered that sexual transmission could have been a source of transmission since John, although in a monogamous relationship at the present, had engaged in unprotected sex while on holiday in the Caribbean four months earlier. The young woman living with John also tested positive for the hepatitis B virus.

Fact from Fiction

Jaundice (latin term is *icterus*) is a symptom not a disease. It brings about a yellowish tinge to a patient's skin color, however it is best recognized on the sclera— the normally white part of the eyes. The yellow pigment bilirubin results from the breakdown of hemoglobin in senescent red blood cells. In liver disease bilirubin binds to connective tissue and stains it yellow.

Fortunately bilirubin is bound to albumin (large plasma protein) in blood and as a result is not able to cross the blood-brain barrier. This means that the brains cells, the grey matter in the hemispheres is not normally stained and damaged. Hepatic encephalopathy however, can occur late in the disease process of fullmanent viral hepatitis and liver cirrhoris.

In general, with viral hepatitis, jaundice is usually of short duration, whereas in liver cirrhosis it is more persistant and chronic. Jaundice may also be accompanied by pruritis (itching).

Yellow skin can also come from hypercaritenemia. The yellow pigment carotene is found in carrots, squash, mangos, and other yellow fruits and vegetables. If a steady diet of foods high in carotene were maintained it could cause yellowing of the skin.

Answer Key & Rationale

1. b) Cirrhosis of the liver is chronic disease with a history of predisposing illnesses including chronic alcoholism, pancreatitis, and hepatitis. The normal liver cells are replaced over time by fibrous bands of connective tissue, which eventually constrict and partition the organ into irregular nodules.

Cholecystitis is an inflammation of the gallbladder, and does not commonly contribute to cirrhosis.

2. d) Tylenol is a trade name for the substance acetaminophen. Acetaminophen is an antipyretic and analgesic. Detoxification takes place in the liver, and overdose can ultimately result in liver failure. Aspirin is a trade name for the substance salicylate (acetylsalicylic acid). Overdose adversely affects all major organ systems as an acid/base imbalance is generated.

3. c) Hepatitis A, also called infectious or short-incubation hepatitis, is spread by saliva, contaminated food and water, as well as feces through poor hygiene. Hepatitis A does not normally lead to chronic hepatitis or cirrhosis. Most patients recover within six to ten weeks and acquire immunity to the virus.

4. a) Hepatitis B, also called serum or long-incubation hepatitis, can be transmitted perinatally and through intimate sexual relations, needle sticks, and intravenous drug use (sharing contaminated needles). Although once believed to be transmitted only through contaminated blood it can also be contacted through human secretions and feces. Hepatitis B is one of the most serious forms of hepatitis, and can lead to cirrhosis, liver cancer, and death. About 1 percent of all cases result in fulminant hepatitis leading to hepatic coma and death usually within two weeks.

5. c) Hepatitis C, formerly called post-transfusion non-A, non-B hepatitis, was formerly undetectable in banked blood, so it was more easily transmitted through transfusions. The route of transmission is parenteral and sexual contact. There is no vaccine for hepatitis C, D, and E.

6. d) Hepatitis D (delta virus) is a co-infection with hepatitis B and is transmitted the same way. As with hepatitis B, the delta virus can lead to active chronic hepatitis and can be fatal. It accounts for about 50 percent of cases with fulminant hepatitis. Type D is usually confined to people who are frequently exposed to blood and blood products, such as IV drug users and hemophiliacs. There is no vaccine for hepatitis E, and, like hepatitis A, it rarely causes death.

7. b); **8.** e); **9.** d) Signs and symptoms commonly associated with Hepatitis B include fever, fatigue, anorexia, malaise, nausea, vomiting, headache, myalgia, and arthralgia in the prodromal (preicteric) stage. Dark-colored urine, light- or clay-colored stools, abdominal pain (particularly the RUQ), a tender, enlarged liver, and jaundice in the second phase. The final phase is the recovery (posticteric) stage, where symptoms subside usually over two to twelve weeks, although sometimes longer. Interestingly, there is often a loss of taste for coffee and cigarettes among those who regularly consume these substances, since there may be changes in the senses of taste and smell.

10. a) Patients with either hepatitis A or B can transmit the infection during the later part of the incubation period before the onset of symptoms. The incubation period for hepatitis A is roughly 15 to 45 days, while hepatitis B is 40 to 180 days.

11. c) Hepatitis B becomes chronic in 5 to 10 percent of cases and is closely associated with liver cancer. Hepatitis B if it reaches the fulminant stage also has a relatively high mortality rate. While many patients go on to become carriers with Hepatitis B, there is no carrier state or chronicity associated with Hepatitis A.

12. a) A vaccine is available for hepatitis B and A (all health care workers should be vaccinated for hepatitis B). There is, however, no vaccine for hepatitis C (although promising research and testing is currently under way). Using gloves and hand washing after contact are part of the standard BSI precautions that should be adhered to when dealing with all patients. Once precautions are taken, the paramedic should not avoid normal patient contact with respect to physical assessment, taking vital signs, assisting or lifting to stretcher, and offering reassurance.

Unless reverse isolation is indicated, the use of a face mask is not a requirement for hepatitis.

CASE STUDY 2

The time was 20:20 hrs. when dispatch received a 911 call from a restaurant in the downtown area. The ambulance crew had just completed a fairly routine transfer, taking an elderly woman from the observation section of the emergency department to her nursing home.

"Twenty-year-old female in seizure" was the information provided, so the crew responded with lights and siren to the emergency. Like all good crews they prepared themselves mentally for what they might expect. They discussed the possibilities and the likelihood that if it was a seizure their patient would most probably be in the postictal phase by the time they arrived.

The dining portion of the restaurant was down a narrow flight of stairs. Their patient, a young woman, was being supported at her head by a friend. The most obvious feature on observation was extreme diaphoresis. She was not in a convulsion on arrival, although witnesses did describe what could be characterized as tremulousness (shaking) lasting two to three minutes.

Her name was Katya. This information came from her friend, since Katya's own responses were somewhat slurred and difficult to understand. On appearance, Katya looked weak and exhausted. She was visibly irritated when asked questions and did not apparently grasp the significance of what was taking place (i.e. that she was obviously not well and in need of assistance). She denied any complaints about pain, except for a pounding headache.

An overview gathered from her friends at the table revealed that they were celebrating following a volleyball tournament that had taken place that day. They were members of the local women's volleyball league, and Katya was one of their newer members, having recently immigrated from Hungary. They denied any knowledge of her medical background and stated that they had just been drinking a couple of glasses of wine and had ordered dinner, which had yet to arrive, when Katya complained of a headache and collapsed. "We just thought it was the wine at first" her friends said, "she appeared drunk, but then she started shaking all over like in a seizure, so we called 911."

Physical exam revealed cool, clammy, pale skin, and a tachycardic pulse. Respirations revealed tachypnea, and her blood pressure was 128/86. Neurological assessment revealed confusion, lethargy, pupils that were dilated but equal and responsive, and grip strength that was weaker on the right side. Her friends said she had a pronounced accent at the best of times, and now she was slurring her words when responding to questions, so that she was virtually impossible to understand.

There were no signs of head trauma (no evidence of hematoma, Battle's sign or periorbital ecchymosis, no rhinorrhea, and no otorrhea), and no history of trauma or recent involvement in a car accident, according to her friends. A quick visual check showed no indication of external bleeding and no apparent sign of incontinence, which is often associated with epileptic seizures. A MedicAlert® bracelet found on her ankle during this assessment identified Katya as a diabetic. Despite this discovery, she denied having any history of illness: epilepsy, allergies, and diabetes included.

There were no medications found in her possession. Her friend examined Katya's wallet but found no additional information.

Suspecting possible hypoglycemia, the EMTs did a finger prick glucose test and found her blood glucose level to be 30 mg/dL. Normal is 70–120 mg/dL. Since Katya was still conscious, the paramedic tried to give her a highly concentrated glucose solution in the form of an oral gel. Suction was close at hand in case she vomited, and her airway was closely monitored. Katya resisted taking the oral glucose and it became clear she was not going to improve on her own. A high concentration of oxygen was also given to offset cerebral hypoxia. An IV of normal saline was initiated and a bolus of 50 percent Dextrose (D50) was administered. If Katya resisted the IV start, the paramedic was prepared to administer 1.0 mg of Glucagon (a hormone that stimulates glycogenolysis in the liver) subcutaneously.

In addition, she was kept warm with blankets and placed semi-prone on the stretcher. Katya was uncooperative to the point of obstinacy at the introduction of each new procedure. However, the attendants' patience, reassurance, and calm voices managed to gain her confidence. After repeated explanations and reasons, she eventually acquiesced, allowing herself to be helped. Within minutes of the administration of the D50 bolus, Katya's level of consciousness and her ability to speak noticeably improved. She admitted her diabetic history and stated that she had simply gone too long without food. She agreed to transport to the hospital and the remainder of the transport was uneventful.

Multiple-Choice Questions

1. Ketoacidosis is normally associated with which of the following?
   1. hypoglycemia
   2. hyperglycemia
   3. decreased ketone levels
   4. increased free fatty acids

      a) 1, 3
      b) 2, 4
      c) 1, 4
      d) 2, 3
      e) 1, 3, 4

2. Precipitating factors related to hypoglycemia can include:
   1. medication error—excessive insulin dose
   2. eating excessively large meals
   3. alcohol consumption without carbohydrate intake
   4. a pancreatic tumor
   5. a general lack of exercise

      a) 1, 2, 3
      b) 2, 3, 5
      c) 1, 4, 5
      d) 2, 4, 5
      e) 1, 3, 4

3. Many patients who are first diagnosed with diabetes mellitus commonly present with:
   1. polyuria
   2. dysuria
   3. polydipsia
   4. polyphagia
   5. dysphagia
   6. dyspnea

      a) 1, 3, 4
      b) 1, 4, 5
      c) 2, 3, 5
      d) 2, 4, 6
      e) 1, 3, 6

4. Complications most often associated with diabetes include:

1. neuropathy
2. vascular disease
3. retinopathy
4. cancer
5. persistent infections
6. osteopathy

   a) 1, 3, 6
   b) 2, 4, 6
   c) 1, 2, 3, 5
   d) 2, 4, 5, 6
   e) 1, 3, 4, 5

5. Signs and symptoms commonly associated with hypoglycemia include:

1. headache
2. diaphoresis
3. fever (pyrexia)
4. tremulousness

   a) 1, 2, 3
   b) 1, 2, 4
   c) 1, 3, 4
   d) 2, 3, 4
   e) all of the above

6. Signs and symptoms commonly associated with hypoglycemia include:

1. Kussmaul's respiration
2. appearance of intoxication
3. confusion and/or irritability
4. hypotension

   a) 1, 3
   b) 2, 3
   c) 1, 2, 4
   d) 1, 3, 4
   e) 2, 3, 4

7. Signs and symptoms commonly associated with hyperglycemia include:

1. cold, clammy skin
2. dehydration
3. decreased pulse pressure
4. tachycardia

   a) 1, 2, 4
   b) 1, 2, 3
   c) 1, 3, 4
   d) 2, 3, 4
   e) all of the above

8. Signs and symptoms commonly associated with ketoacidosis include:

1. dry warm skin
2. garlic breath odor
3. Kussmaul's respiration
4. hypotension

    a) 1, 3, 4
    b) 1, 2, 4
    c) 2, 3, 4
    d) 1, 2, 3
    e) all of the above

9. Alcohol consumption by an individual with diabetes will have which of the following effects?

    a) increased glycogenolysis
    b) inhibition of gluconeogenesis
    c) increased gluconeogenesis
    d) inhibition of glycogenolysis
    e) none of the above

10. Which of the following statements concerning hypoglycemia is/are true?

1. The onset of signs and symptoms is generally rapid, often occurring within minutes.
2. If conscious, the patient will always be able to relate a history of taking insulin.
3. If a gag reflex is absent, sugar liquids should be given anyway since the chance of coma and irreversible brain damage is great.
4. Oral hypoglycemic agents will help to minimize the risk of a decreasing level of consciousness.

    a) 1
    b) 1, 2
    c) 2, 4
    d) 1, 3, 4
    e) 2, 3, 4

11. In differentiating insulin-dependent and non–insulin-dependent diabetics, which of the following are correct?

1. Insulin-dependent diabetics comprise the majority of diabetics.
2. Non–insulin-dependent diabetics are more likely to be over forty years of age.
3. Insulin-dependent diabetics are more likely to have a long history of obesity.
4. Non–insulin-dependent diabetics are more likely to be ketosis resistant.

    a) 1, 2

    b) 2, 3
    c) 2, 4
    d) 1, 4
    e) 1, 3

12. Ketoacidosis, which can be an acute complication of diabetes, is often associated with the following:

    1. infection, fever
    2. stress, trauma
    3. Kussmaul's respiration
    4. nausea, vomiting

        a) 1, 2, 3
        b) 1, 2, 4
        c) 1, 3, 4
        d) 2, 3, 4
        e) all of the above

Debriefing

This call, like so many others, was received just after the completion of a non-emergency transfer. It is not always easy to make the quick transition and to anticipate all that is necessary in responding to an emergency.

Dispatchers have a difficult job at best. The information provided to them most often comes from a non-professional (a friend or a relative of the patient) who is under a great deal of stress. Prehospital providers should always keep an open mind regarding the true nature of the emergency while responding to the call.

While most seizure-related calls involve epilepsy, there are many that involve a wide variety of other problems, including hypoglycemia. In this case the classic phases of a seizure, including the postictal phase discussed by the EMTs en route, would not be part of the picture.

It is important to keep an open mind, but it is even more important to review, at least to oneself, the alternate possibilities that could arise. A restaurant scene demands special attention because cafe coronaries (choking on food bolus) or possibly anaphylactic shock from a food allergy can both be life-threatening emergencies where immediate action on the part of the EMTs may make all the difference.

Fortunately, Katya was not choking, nor was she experiencing severe dyspnea. She had not yet eaten, and although the sulfa product in most wines can, for some, produce an allergic reaction, there was no burning or tightness in her chest, no rash or flushed appearance. In fact, she was somewhat pale.

Could the alcohol alone be the cause of Katya's problems? Indeed, working as hard as she had by playing volleyball in a competition, combined with very little food intake, may have increased the intoxicating effect of alcohol, but alcohol is a vasodilator and would produce a flushed appearance rather than the pale diaphoretic skin condition seen in Katya. Signs similar to inebriation may be mistaken for alcohol intoxication; however, there are a number of underlying pathologies where confusion, slurred speech, and a decreasing level of consciousness (LOC) are present. Accurate history taking and a thorough secondary assessment are essential in moving beyond what seems obvious to the untrained eye.

Alcohol may well have contributed to Katya's hypoglycemia since alcohol helps prevent glycogenolysis, the break down of glycogen (glucose stored in the liver in the form of a starch) to glucose.

Due to Katya's low blood glucose level, her body has responded with an exaggerated epinephrine response. Epinephrine released from the adrenal medulla stimulates muscle cells and liver cells to break down glycogen. Diaphoresis, dilated pupils, tachycardia, tachypnea, paleness, and trembling can all be attributed to this massive adrenaline release.

The brain relies almost exclusively on glucose as its source of energy, which it stores in adenosine triphosphate (ATP). A shortfall in supply will result in almost immediate cerebral dysfunction. This is called neuroglycopenia and is characterized by confusion, headache, and fatigue. If left untreated, cerebral hypoxia can induce unconsciousness with coma and possibly permanent CNS damage not long afterwards. Katya's denial of being a diabetic, despite her MedicAlert® bracelet, is not unusual for someone in a hypoglycemic state because of the associated confusion and disorientation. It should be remembered that many well-meaning patients may deny relevant past medical histories in the presence of a decreased LOC. Interestingly, most known epileptics will also deny any history of their disease in the early postictal phase of a seizure. At the same time, convulsions are not uncommon during episodes of hypoglycemia.

Finally, because of the effect on the CNS, hypoglycemia may mimic the signs of a stroke. Katya's slurred speech and right-sided paresis may be mistaken for the signs of a left-sided cerebrovascular accident (CVA), but not when the whole picture is taken into account.

Follow-Up

Katya's vital signs were monitored on the way to hospital and within ten minutes of the administration of the D50 she accepted a package of glucose gel. Her blood glucose level was re-evaluated and found to be 94. Her neurological status showed dramatic improvement. Katya was able to relate that she indeed was an insulin-dependent diabetic. She had not eaten since breakfast and was about to get up and get a chocolate bar, which she had in her windbreaker, when she started feeling strange. She then collapsed and became confused.

Upon arrival at the hospital, her blood sugar levels were monitored. The emergency department diagnosis was hypoglycemia secondary to insulin reaction. After a short stay, which included a review of her regimen, Katya was released and was even able to work out with her volleyball team the following day.

Fact from Fiction

Diabetes mellitus comes from the Greek "to pass through" and "sweat" which refers to two main signs and indications for the disease—polyuria and glycosuria.

Glucose in the blood is regulated by the hormones insulin and glucagon, which are secreted from the beta cells and alpha cells respectively and located in the islets if Langerhans within the pancreas. Destruction of the beta cells will lead to diabetes mellitus and the classic sign of hyperglycemia. In addition, since insulin facilitates transport of glucose from the blood to the tissues, an increase in tissue resistance owing to faulty insulin receptors or antibodies to insulin can also lead to or contribute to diabetes mellitus.

Another form of diabetes is called diabetes insipidus. It is caused by pituitary disease and does not produce glycosuria. In ancient times physicians tested urine by licking it with their fingers and diagnosing diabetes mellitus if the urine was sweet or diabetes insipidus if the urine was tasteless. Insipid in Latin means "without taste."

Answer Key & Rationale

1. b) Ketoacidosis represents a state of metabolic acidosis secondary to hyperglycemia in insulin-dependent diabetics. A lack of insulin, necessary to transport glucose into the body's cells, results in a search for alternative fuels. Glucose is left to accumulate in the blood stream while fats are broken down (a process known as lipolysis) into triglyceride and fatty acids to be used by the cells to create energy. The waste by-products are called ketones or keto acids, which increase the amount of metabolic acids in the bloodstream, hence the name ketoacidosis.

2. e) Hypoglycemia, or low blood glucose, most often results from medication error. Insulin is the transporter of glucose into the body's cell and there exists a fine line between supply and demand. Too much insulin means blood sugar levels in the vascular system will drop. Alcohol consumption can also contribute to low levels of blood glucose by blocking glycogenolysis (breakdown of glycogen to glucose). Glycogen is stored in the liver and is available to be broken down into glucose if blood sugar levels drop. Alcohol prevents glycogen breakdown and may consequently exacerbate a state of hypoglycemia. A pancreatic tumor has been known to result in the release of an excessive amount of insulin leading to hypoglycemia. It is important to keep an open mind, however, since other pathologies may also lead to hypoglycemia, such as hypopituitarism, hypoadrenalism, neural and liver disease.

A lack of exercise decreases the cells' demand for glucose, while eating large meals only adds to an increase in blood glucose. This increase requires more insulin (which, among its other tasks, helps store the excess glucose). A prolonged binge on sweets and junk food, on the other hand, can lead to large fluctuations in blood glucose levels, which may result in what is known as rebound hypoglycemia.

3. a) Polyuria, polydipsia, and polyphagia are the three cardinal signs of diabetes mellitus. They stem from a prolonged rise in blood glucose levels, the result of an insufficient amount of insulin being secreted by the pancreas. A hyperosmolarity is created in the vascular system by the glucoses not being transported into the body's cells. Water from tissue cells is drawn into the vascular system to compensate for the unequal concentration gradient and is then released through the kidneys. The result leads to excessive urination (polyuria), dehydration, and excessive thirst (polydipsia). Since the body's cells are starved for glucose, despite all the glucose in the vascular system, the person is also constantly hungry (polyphagia).

Dysuria refers to painful or difficult urination, while dysphagia is difficult or painful swallowing and dyspnea is painful or difficult respirations.

4. c) There are possibly more complications arising from diabetes than any other disease, not the least of which is the vascular disease arteriosclerosis, which leads to myocardial infarction and cerebrovascular accidents. Retinopathy among diabetics is one of the major causes of blindness. There are numerous forms of neurological complications including peripheral neuropathy (which is usually compounded with vascular occlusion resulting in ulcers), particularly of the feet. Since the immune system is also compromised in the diabetic as a result of increased blood glucose levels, infections are quite common and a lack of adequate protein (the result of using alternate fuels, which include protein as well as fat) means that healing will take much longer among diabetics.

While cancers and osteopathy may well be seen among diabetics, they are not considered direct complications.

5. b); **6.** b) Signs and symptoms of hypoglycemia include tachycardia, diaphoresis, pallor, fatigue, tremulousness, irritability, headache, diplopia, and confusion progressing to somnolence and ultimately coma. The confusion, a result of neuroglycopenia, may be mistaken for alcohol intoxication. Personality changes, also related to the lack of glucose for brain cells, may be seen in some patients. As well, cerebral hypoxia may result in seizure activity in some cases.

7. d); **8.** a) Signs and symptoms of hyperglycemia include tachycardia, decreased blood pressure (decreased pulse pressure in particular), warm dry skin and poor skin turgor (signs of dehydration), fever, polyuria, polydipsia, and polyphagia. When an insulin-dependent diabetic suffers from hyperglycemia, the additional signs of ketoacidosis may be present. These include Kussmaul's respiration; a fruity or acetone breath odor, the result of a build up of ketones; hyperventilation in order to compensate for metabolic acidosis by blowing off carbon dioxide; nausea and vomiting due to the increase in acidity. In addition, a decreasing LOC will gradually occur, since metabolic acidosis leads to CNS depression.

9. d) Alcohol prevents the breakdown of glycogen stores in the liver. The result is an increased risk of hypoglycemia when the diabetic consumes alcohol. Glycogenolysis is the process of creating glucose from glycogen; alcohol interrupts this process. Those at greatest risk are chronic alcohol abusers who tend to eat poorly and have very little glycogen in reserve. Unfortunately, hypoglycemia may be mistaken for inebriation (drunkenness), delaying treatment.

10. a) Since the brain uses glucose almost to the exclusion of all other fuels, a deficit in glucose brings the signs and symptoms of hypoglycemia in rapid order. Hyperglycemia, on the other hand, with its subsequent buildup of metabolic acidosis, occurs gradually over hours or perhaps even days.

Confusion and disorientation resulting from hypoglycemia does not always allow the patient to relate an accurate history. If a gag reflex is absent, and the patient insufficiently conscious, then introducing fluids of any kind could induce aspiration which may severely compromise the airway, and is thus contraindicated. Oral hypoglycemic agents are medication in the form of pills designed to enhance whatever production of insulin is still available in non–insulin-dependent diabetics and would consequently not be of benefit to a hypoglycemic patient. Sugar, glucose, and dextrose, if taken orally, would all benefit a conscious hypoglycemic patient.

11. c) Non–insulin-dependent diabetics have a mismatch in insulin production and energy needs. They are still capable of producing insulin but not enough to meet their needs. They comprise the majority of diabetics, are usually over forty when diagnosed, and often carry more weight than is normal for their age. Since some insulin production is still available to the non–insulin-dependent diabetic, the effects of ketoacidosis during states of hyperglycemia are usually prevented.

12. e) Hyperglycemia, with the ensuing ketoacidosis in insulin-dependent diabetics, can be precipitated by stress, trauma, infection, or illness. These
states result in an increase in energy needs and therefore require a similar
increase in insulin. Not taking insulin, overeating, and lack of exercise
may also contribute to the clinical picture of hyperglycemia. Kussmaul's
respiration is an attempt by the body to compensate for metabolic acidosis. The pneumotaxic center in the brain detects an increase in acidity (the
accumulation of keto acids) and increases the rate and depth of respirations in order to compensate by blowing off carbon dioxide, which is
itself an acid. This is an attempt at decreasing the overall acidity of the
blood. Nausea and vomiting may also occur when the acidosis persists.
Vomiting can contribute to overall dehydration and ultimately hypovolemic shock, which may develop as a result of osmotic diuresis.

CASE STUDY 3

Dusk covered the city. The sun had disappeared, but the sky refused to give up and clung to a pale gray-blue. The last of the commuters, those who had worked the longest day, were finally on their way home. The approach of evening carried a warm breeze sweeping over the last remnants of snow banks. Suddenly, reality jarred its way into the stationary ambulance on standby, via the radio: MVA motorcycle/car, multiple patients, unknown injuries.

For the prehospital EMS providers, nothing marks the change of seasons as sharply as the appearance of motorcycles in spring.

As the ambulance neared the scene, two circles of bystanders were forming in the intersection. The police had just arrived and were controlling traffic and moving people back. The ambulance crew was directed to two patients lying 30 feet apart. One was an adult male showing no signs of movement. The other was a young boy, conscious and obviously in pain.

The EMTs quickly ascertained that the adult was pulseless and non-breathing. With the help of an off-duty firefighter, that patient's motorcycle helmet was removed, an airway established using the modified jaw thrust maneuver, an oral-pharyngeal airway inserted, and while the fireman initiated cardiac compressions, the paramedic set up the oxygen and commenced ventilation (bagging). The patient was also quickly intubated.

The police officer, when questioned, informed the crew that there were just the two victims; the single occupant of the minivan, which had collided with the motorcycle, was not complaining of any injuries. Witnesses described the accident to police as a rear-end collision. The motorcycle had been stopped and was about to make a left turn when it was struck from behind. The speed of the minivan was estimated at between twenty-five and thirty miles an hour. The passenger on the motorcycle was thrown approximately twenty feet while the driver received the impact and skidded to a halt with his bike.

The passenger of the motorcycle was lying with a leg in a severely angulated position, revealing an obvious fracture of the right lower leg. The victim was a young male, conscious and yelling about the pain he was experiencing in his leg. The second paramedic quickly conducted a primary assessment. From the boy's loud yelling, he concluded that the airway was well established. Then the EMT made sure his patient did not move, particularly with respect to his head: a smooth bike helmet can easily roll from side to side.

The passenger's name was Justin, and he knew where he was but did not remember being hit or thrown. He had no complaint of breathing difficulty, and a visual inspection revealed no obvious chest trauma or asymmetrical movement. He had a strong radial pulse, and a quick hands-on check for bleeding revealed a large blood-soaked area just below the right knee. The paramedic cut Justin's jeans to expose a compound tibia and possibly fibula fracture. There were bone fragments, which could be seen through the skin. A large bulky sterile dressing produced from the trauma kit was laid over the area and secured with roller gauze. Assessment of the area revealed a pale foot, absent pedal pulses, delayed capillary refill, no sensation, and an inability to move the toes.

During assessment the paramedic had a bystander remain at Justin's head to ensure immobility and to maintain verbal contact. Justin's only complaint was of severe pain. However, this pain was not in his right leg as first thought, but in his left just below the knee. Exposure of his left leg revealed ecchymosis over the calf, pain and tenderness to palpation, and extreme pain on flexion of the toes. Distal circulation, however, appeared to be good.

By this time, after almost five minutes at the scene, a second ambulance arrived. The patient with CPR in progress was provided with a cervical collar, had all of his clothes removed, rolled as a unit onto a backboard, secured in place, and connected to a cardiac monitor/defibrillator. The monitor showed asystole apart from the manual compressions, and no defibrillation was indicated. Multiple large-bore IVs were quickly inserted. He was quickly placed on the stretcher and moved to one of the two ambulances. The police officer had retrieved the victim's wallet and identified him as thirty-six-year-old Roger Riopelle. The firefighter volunteered to help continue CPR en route, and Roger was taken to the nearest emergency department.

Realizing that there was no problem that justified immediate removal of Justin's helmet, the paramedic decided to remove it anyway, to allow immediate and complete airway access if it became necessary. Justin had his helmet removed with the help of the second crew member, and a quick assessment revealed an absence of visible head or neck injury. A cervical collar was, nonetheless, secured in place. He was placed on a high concentration of oxygen, and the right leg was straightened and splinted. Immobilization would have been impractical as the leg initially lay, since it would not have accommodated the stretcher. The paramedic also hoped there might be some restoration of distal circulation, but a subsequent neurovascular assessment revealed no change. Justin, who remained conscious and alert as he was immobilized to a spinal board, began asking for his dad. The paramedic replied that his dad had also been injured in the accident but was being cared for and taken to the hospital. While the paramedic kept him talking, Justin revealed that he would be eleven next week, and that he had no previous medical history. The paramedic briefly considered implementation of their pain management protocol, but due to the close proximity to the hospital, he decided against it. Justin was secured to the stretcher and placed inside the ambulance where a large-bore IV line was started with lactated Ringer's solution.

Additional assessment en route revealed no evidence of tenderness, instability, or hematomas to the head or neck; trachea was midline; palpation of ribs revealed no tenderness, and good excursion; palpation of abdominal quadrants showed no evidence of tenderness, rigidity, guarding, or distention; pain and instability were demonstrated when the pelvis was palpated; and the upper legs and arms revealed no evidence of injury.

A radial pulse continued to be rapid and strong while Justin's LOC showed no sign of deterioration. The Children's Hospital was alerted to the arrival of an eleven-year-old male, conscious and alert with possible pelvic and compound tib/fib fractures; the mechanism of injury the result of a motorcycle/car collision.

As Justin was being moved into the emergency department, his condition quickly deteriorated, seemingly without warning. He stopped talking, and became extremely pale, with a weak and thready pulse, and obvious tachypnea.

Multiple-Choice Questions

1. According to national statistics, which of the following statements are true?
   1. Trauma is the leading cause of death in North America between the ages of one and forty-four.
   2. Children in the age group one to fourteen are twice as likely to die as the result of accidents than from any other cause.
   3. Twenty percent of all deaths in the age group fifteen to twenty-four are caused by motor vehicle accidents.
   4. Overall, trauma is the third leading cause of death.

      a) 1, 4
      b) 2, 4
      c) 1, 3, 4
      d) 2, 3, 4
      e) all of the above

2. In understanding the kinematics of trauma, certain laws of physics (the study of interaction between energy and matter) must also be understood. Which statements are correct?

  1. Newton's first law of motion states that gravity creates a positive energy affecting all bodies.
  2. A second law of physics states that energy cannot be created or destroyed, but can only change form.
  3. A car striking another vehicle causes kinetic energy to be transformed into mechanical energy.
  4. Kinetic energy reveals speed to be a greater influence on transmitted energy than weight.

    a) 1, 2, 3
    b) 1, 2, 4
    c) 1, 3, 4
    d) 2, 3, 4
    e) all of the above

3. Risk of death is increased _____ times by those victims of motor vehicle accidents who are ejected from their vehicle because they failed to wear a lap and shoulder harness.

  a) 5
  b) 10
  c) 50
  d) 100
  e) 300

4. The "golden hour" refers to the sixty-minute period after trauma is sustained, during which it is crucial to get critically injured patients to definitive care, including surgical intervention if required. During the golden hour

  1. rapid assessment and treatment of the chief complaint should be the only concern at scene.
  2. ideally, ten minutes is the maximum amount of time to be on scene with a severely injured trauma patient.
  3. all multisystem trauma patients of motor vehicle accidents must receive spinal immobilization.
  4. in situations of significant trauma the secondary survey (comprehensive head to toe assessment) must be carried out on scene.

    a) 1, 2
    b) 2, 3
    c) 1, 4
    d) 2, 3, 4
    e) 1, 3, 4

5. Motor vehicle accidents often involve fractures, which may initially show the following signs and symptoms:

1. point tenderness
2. pitting edema
3. deformity
4. loss of movement
5. loss of proximal pulse

   a) 1, 2, 3
   b) 1, 4, 5
   c) 2, 3, 5
   d) 1, 3, 4
   e) 2, 4, 5

6. Signs and symptoms of fractures may include:

1. paresthesia
2. crepitation
3. loss of sensation
4. delayed capillary refill
5. pallor

   a) 1, 2, 4
   b) 1, 3, 5
   c) 1, 2, 3, 4
   d) 2, 3, 4, 5
   e) all of the above

7. Trauma that results in compound fractures may risk which of the following complications?

1. vascular impairment
2. fat embolus
3. osteomyelitis
4. compartment syndrome
5. osteoporosis
6. sepsis
7. peripheral nerve damage

   a) 1, 2, 4, 5
   b) 2, 3, 5, 6
   c) 1, 4, 6, 7
   d) 1, 2, 3, 6, 7
   e) 1, 3, 4, 5, 7

8. Trauma to children may result in hypovolemia from hemorrhage involving large bone fractures. The earliest sign(s) of hypovolemia in children are usually manifested in:

a) pallor and coolness
b) hypotension
c) bradycardia
d) hyperventilation
e) decreased LOC

9. Differentiate between the normal vital signs of children and those of adults:

1. Respiratory rates increase with age.
2. Pulse rates decrease with age.
3. Blood pressure increases with age.
4. Skin condition becomes more reliable with age.

    a) 1, 4
    b) 2, 3
    c) 2, 4
    d) 1, 2, 3
    e) 1, 3, 4

10. Which of the following statements relating to children and shock are true?

1. Hypovolemia is the most common cause.
2. Compensatory mechanisms are weak.
3. Orthostatic vital signs are a good indicator.
4. Deterioration is constant and progressive.
5. Small amounts of fluid loss can be catastrophic.

    a) 1, 2, 3
    b) 2, 3, 5
    c) 1, 3, 5
    d) 1, 2, 4
    e) 3, 4, 5

11. Management of children with multisystem trauma leading to shock includes:

1. high concentration oxygen
2. spinal immobilization
3. fluid challenge
4. maintenance of body heat
5. elevating extremities
6. constant reassurance

    a) 1, 3, 4, 6
    b) 2, 3, 5, 6

    c) 1, 2, 3, 4, 5
    d) 1, 2, 4, 5, 6
    e) all of the above

12. Complications resulting from uncompensated hypovolemic shock include:
1. hepatic failure
2. coagulopathy
3. renal failure
4. metabolic alkalosis
5. cardiovascular collapse

    a) 1, 2, 4
    b) 2, 3, 5
    c) 1, 3, 4, 5
    d) 1, 2, 3, 5
    e) all of the above

Debriefing

Late afternoon into early evening is a precarious time of day for driving. People are often tired and still wrapped up in the day's events, yet anxious to get home and unwind. On the physical side, the axial skeleton has lost almost two centimeters in height over the course of the day so that car mirrors may be improperly adjusted, increasing the danger to motorcyclists who are not driving the most obvious vehicles on the road.

The arrival of spring adds a new dimension to driving with the advent of motorbikes and cyclists on the road. While motorcycles are obviously much smaller than other vehicles, they are capable of the same speed; cyclists necessitate an increased awareness for the space on the right side of the road. The need for vigilance seems to increase overnight, as if all two-wheel drivers decide collectively on the same day to dust off their bikes. No matter how well motorcycle and bicycle riders obey the rules of the road, there will be occasions when they are simply not seen or when someone is not paying attention to them. The result is often disastrous for those on a vehicle which offers no outside protection.

Prehospital professionals should assume that victims of motorcycle and bicycle accidents have multisystem trauma until evidence proves otherwise. The cervical spine should automatically receive immobilization. The thoracic and lumbar spine get at least a little support from the ribs and torso respectively, and a helmet provides protection for the head, but the cervical spine is completely exposed. It is little wonder that most spinal cord injuries occur between C2 and C7.

Internal injuries including hemorrhage should also be suspected, particularly when the force, speed, and distance thrown indicate considerable energy transmitted. A simple tib/fib or radius/ulna fracture may be the only complaint from the patient, but if a fractured pelvis or a lacerated spleen, liver, pancreas, kidney, or lung coexist, the patient is at risk for hypovolemic shock.

When assessing potential injury, it is important to look at the damage sustained by the vehicles involved, and remember that the patients have been subjected to the same forces. Also, when reporting potential injury to emergency staff at hospital, remember that they have not had the benefit of viewing the scene and seeing the damage to vehicles; therefore, they need a clear picture including direction, speed, and mass.

$$\text{Kinetic energy} = \frac{\text{mass (weight)} \times \text{velocity (speed)}^2}{2}$$

The interesting factor in this equation is velocity, for if the speed is doubled, the amount of kinetic energy produced quadruples. The saying "speed kills" is not without merit.

Also note the direction of contact, head on, lateral, rear, rotational, or rollover. These factors may all provide clues as to the nature of injuries sustained.

Multisystem trauma requires definitive care within the hour, which may necessitate a compromise in completing full on-scene assessments. The total time at scene should be limited to ten minutes or less. Never compromise on safety, however. Running motors, engine fires, gasoline leaks, and so on, deserve immediate attention. The primary survey, concentrating on airway management with spinal control, ventilation with oxygen, and circulation with hemorrhage control is essential to patient care. Subsequent assessment and treatment of the chief complaint, followed by rapid transport, should take precedence over a comprehensive head-to-toe assessment and additional vital signs, which may have to be conducted en route.

Despite the time constraints, information gathering should continue throughout trauma scenarios and should be as complete as possible. A patient's medical history may uncover a blood dyscrasia such as hemophilia or a medication such as Coumadin, warfarin, or heparin (anticoagulants); these discoveries may significantly alter the potential severity and speed of onset to shock.

In determining the chief complaint, it is important to keep in mind that hypovolemia may often be hidden when it is the result of internal hemorrhage. Massive bleeding can result from a pelvic fracture, which may show little evidence of swelling or deformity. The paramedic should examine the patient for pelvic tenderness or instability. Note: extremity fractures of the femur and tib/fib should not receive traction in the presence of an unstable pelvis. The best treatment for all fractures is immobilization (traction is one common method of immobilization; the term refers to the maintenance of an in-line force and does not constitute reduction, the actual realignment of bones). Despite the premium placed on time in situations of major trauma, all immobilization should include both a pre- and post-neurovascular assessment distal to the site of injury.

As this case shows, children are not simply smaller versions of adults. They need special consideration in situations of trauma. It is prudent to remember the saying "sitting pretty one minute and going downhill the next." Children may initially appear to be "sitting pretty" because the cardiovascular system in children is much more adaptive than that in adults. Heart rates are higher, blood vessels are more elastic, and there is a greater response from the release of adrenaline and cortisol to stress. The benefit, however, is strictly short-term. Once decompensation starts, children have very little circulatory reserve. The overall vascular fluid volume is much less than in adults, and a significantly lower blood loss can send a child into profound shock.

Death from trauma can occur in any of the following three time frames. In the first time frame, death takes place within seconds to minutes. This leaves little time to salvage patients because of injury to major vessels and organs such as the aorta, the heart, the brain, brainstem, and spinal cord. In the second time frame, death occurs in minutes to a few hours. Here the paramedic can make all the difference by conducting efficient, competent, and effective assessment, treatment, and transport to definitive care. During this time period, the "golden hour," a patient sustaining multisystem trauma stands a good chance for a full recovery, if provided with definitive care (including surgery) within one hour after injury. In the third time frame, death occurs over days to weeks following injury, and is often the result of organ failure or secondary complications such as sepsis. Complications that arise in this time frame can also be substantially reduced with appropriate prehospital care.

Follow-Up

Justin was found to be in hypovolemic shock with a fractured pelvis, compound (R)tibia/fibula fracture, and compartment syndrome of the (L)soleus. Using the line started by the paramedic en route to the hospital, a fluid challenge of lactated Ringer's solution was administered along with an infusion of whole blood after cross-matching, and Justin was taken to surgery.

Unfortunately, Mr. Riopelle was pronounced dead shortly after arriving in the emergency department. The cause of death was massive internal thoracic injuries leading to cardiac arrest. The injuries included a lacerated aorta and extensive hemothorax resulting in cardiac tamponade and pulseless electrical activity (PEA).

Justin's recovery was obviously complicated by his dad's death. However, although rehabilitation was slow, he progressed well and even managed to make a computer link with his teacher and classmates while in the hospital.

Fact from Fiction

When treating compound or open fractures it is essential to maintain aseptic technique since there is a significant risk of introducing a bacterial infection into the wound. The danger here is that the infection leads to osteomyelitis, which can severely and permanently damage bone.

When a bone is broken there is damage to the periosteum and blood vessels in the cortex, marrow, and surrounding tissue. Bleeding occurs at the break site and a hematoma develops from within the medullary canal and forms between the fractured ends of the bones. Tissue near the break is cut off from adequate perfusion and the resulting ischemia and necrosis brings on an inflammatory response. The presence of inflammatory leukocytes and mast cells, the subsequent release of histamine and resultant vasodilation and edema bring about the warmth, redness, and swollen appearance of the fracture.

Within two days after the injury, repair is well underway. Decalcification of fractured bone ends from osteoclasts, invasion of osteoblasts to synthesis collagen and matrix, callus formation, and finally remodeling to remove excess callus all occur in this regeneration process.

Bone is one of only two body tissues that are able to regenerate; it creates new bone, as opposed to scar tissue, when it heals. The other body tissue able to regenerate is the liver.

Answer Key & Rationale

1. a) In North America, trauma is the leading cause of death from age one up to middle age, and overall it ranks third behind cardiovascular disease and cancers. Children in the age group one to fourteen are four times more likely to die as a result of accidents than from any other cause. Close to 40 percent of all deaths in the age group fifteen to twenty-four are caused by motor vehicle accidents.

2. d) Newton's first law of motion states that a body at rest will remain at rest and a body in motion will remain in motion until acted upon by some outside force. Energy can neither be created nor destroyed but can only change form. Some forms of energy include thermal, electrical, chemical, radiant, and mechanical energy. This last is the form taken when damage is sustained to both car and occupants during motor vehicle collisions.

Kinetic energy is based on a relationship between weight and speed. If, for example, two bullets are fired, the first with twice the mass (weight) as the second but traveling at half the velocity (speed), the second bullet will result in twice the impact energy despite its small size. Velocity, not mass, accounts for the greater percentage of force created.

3. e) When worn properly, a lap and shoulder harness combination reduces morbidity and mortality significantly. Ejection from a vehicle during a collision increases the risk of death 300 times. The restrained occupant is also less likely to have his/her body collide with the inside of the vehicle, further reducing the potential for serious injury.

4. b) While rapid assessment and treatment of the chief complaint is important, the initial priority at any trauma scene is to identify hazards and recognize immediate life-threatening problems in the primary survey. Once these are identified and recognized, attempts should be made to correct them.

Keeping in mind the "golden hour," ten minutes should be the maximum time at scene. Exhaustive head-to-toe secondary assessments may have to await completion en route, time and injuries permitting.

As a matter of protocol, all patients who have sustained traumatic injury in an MVA should receive spinal immobilization as a precautionary measure even if there are no obvious signs or symptoms of cervical injury at the time.

5. d); **6.** e)   Clinical characteristics of fractures include pain, point tenderness, deformity, loss of movement, loss of distal pulse, paresthesia, crepitation, loss of sensation, delayed capillary refill (less than two seconds), and pale skin.

Discoloration (ecchymosis) and swelling often develop over time, but are rarely seen at the time of injury.

When extremities are involved, comparisons should be made with the unaffected limb.

7. d) Complications resulting from fractures include arterial and nerve damage; pulmonary embolus from fat (in marrow) if long bone fractures are involved; and infection from compound (open) fractures that may produce sepsis or osteomyelitis, particularly in children.

A compartment syndrome develops secondary to a contusion often without the presence of a fracture. Ischemia and pain occur as blood vessels have lost their integrity and swelling develops within the layers of facia surrounding muscle fibers.

Osteoporosis is a chronic degenerative loss of bone and may be the primary event to a spontaneous fracture, particularly hip fractures among elderly women.

8. a) Skin which is pale (white), and cold, clammy (diaphoretic) to touch is often the earliest sign of shock in children. Strong compensatory mechanisms serve to maintain cardiac output and blood pressure in the young, as blood is shunted from peripheral skin tissues to the core.

9. b) Vital signs vary with age. Both respiratory and pulse rates decrease with age, whereas blood pressure increases. Preschool children with heart rates over 100 and respiratory rates between 20 and 30 are not abnormal. Normal values, for systolic pressure in children, can be estimated by doubling their age in years and adding 80.

Skin condition becomes a less reliable indicator for shock as a person ages. In the elderly, arteries become less compliant and peripheral circulation is often compromised.

10. c) Hypovolemia is by far the most common cause of shock among children. Fluid and electrolyte loss through dehydration resulting from diarrhea, vomiting, or inadequate fluid intake is often the cause. A reduction in circulating volume can also be the result of internal or external bleeding from trauma.

Compensatory mechanisms, including the release of adrenaline, are very strong in children, and shock may be detected in its early stages by taking orthostatic (postural) vital signs. Increases in heart rate or a reduction in pulse pressure, in a sitting position as opposed to supine, would indicate circulatory compromise.

Outward signs of shock may not be easily seen in children until decompensation starts. Once the line is crossed where compensation no longer provides adequate perfusion, decompensation ensues, with rapidly deteriorating LOC and imminent death.

Because of the size difference, a loss of half a liter of blood may represent only a ten percent loss of total blood volume in an adult, but a twenty to thirty percent loss of circulatory volume in a young child.

11. e) Management of children who have sustained multisystem trauma includes: reassurance and an empathetic approach; spinal immobilization; 100 percent oxygen delivery; intravenous fluids (intraosseous if IV in a vein cannot be established) of lactated Ringer's or normal saline; maintenance of body warmth with blankets; shock position with extremities elevated; and ongoing assessment and monitoring of vital signs.

12. d) Major complications secondary to prolonged perfusion compromise can include organ failure of the heart, lungs, liver, and kidneys. Severe cerebral hypoxia may also result in permanent brain damage. As clotting factors are used up, coagulopathy and gastrointestinal bleeding can complicate prolonged shock. In addition, secondary to poor perfusion and tissue hypoxia, anaerobic metabolism will result in the acid/base imbalance of metabolic acidosis.

CASE STUDY 4

On arrival at the river, the ambulance crew found no patients. Instead, they were met by the fire department rescue squad, who had received a call claiming that two boys were clinging to an ice floe close to shore. It was early spring and the above-zero temperatures during the day were sending large flat blocks of ice floating into the river's main channel.

The sun had just disappeared over the horizon and a powerful fire department spotlight was moving methodically over the surface, searching for the two boys. They were spotted in mid-river about a hundred yards out, drifting on a ten-by-fifteen-foot ice floe. There were no cries or sounds coming from the boys, yet onlookers felt encouraged by some movement on the floe.

The fire department rescue squad had a large inflatable boat with an outboard engine. With the help of all available, it was lowered down a fairly steep embankment into the icy water.

Last-minute instructions to the rescue squad by the EMTs stressed the importance of handling the victims gently, particularly if one was unconscious. The operative words concerning patient contact were "fragile: handle with care." Progress by the rescue squad was slow since the evening temperatures were refreezing the water close to shore. They had to break the ice with oars in order to make headway.

A second ambulance was requested and, in the meantime, the heat in the first ambulance was turned up high and extra blankets were placed next to the heaters in order to warm them. The outside temperature had dropped significantly from earlier in the day and now stood at 20°F (−6°C). A slight northeasterly wind created a wind-chill temperature of 15°F (−11°C).

In a testament to the professionalism of the fire department, the rescue of the boys was successful and without incident.

As the two boys were carried up the embankment to the awaiting stretchers, it was apparent that one of the boys was unconscious. They were placed in the ambulance where the paramedics established that the unresponsive boy did have a faint bradycardic carotid pulse and a shallow respiratory rate of 8 per minute. The patient was quickly intubated and ventilation was assisted with warmed oxygen. His clothes, which were wet and cold, were removed. The paramedics attempted to initiate an IV, but couldn't find a visible or palpable vein. It was noted that neither boy was wearing any kind of hat.

The second boy was conscious and gave his name as David, and said his friend's name was Jason. David, whose upper body was dry, was helped in removing his pants, which were soaked from the knees down. His socks and shoes were drenched in icy cold water and, when removed, revealed cold, pale feet with waxy looking toes, which were without feeling and lacked capillary refill. Pedal pulses were non-palpable and, when asked, the boy was unable to move his toes. David was quickly bundled into one of the pre-warmed blankets and placed into the back of the second ambulance.

David's speech was slow and slurred and hampered by a constant, almost violent shivering. However, the story eventually came to light that he and Jason, both thirteen years old, had been walking along the ice close to shore on the way home from school. Whenever cracks developed in one area, they would leap over the crack to another section. When a particular section gave way and drifted out, the leap to shore quickly became too great for David. He yelled to Jason that he could not swim. Jason, who was on another section, did not wish to abandon his friend, so he jumped into the frigid water and was helped onto the ice floe by David. The distance from shore was less than two meters but the water was literally ice cold, so the boys started yelling for help. Meanwhile, the ice floe drifted steadily toward the river's center.

It was twenty-five minutes before their cries were heard and another forty-five minutes before they were rescued and back on land.

On assessment, Jason's pupils were dilated but reactive to light, although slow to respond. He was pale and cold to the touch, and the removal of his wet clothes was extremely difficult because of pronounced muscular rigidity. His jacket, shirt, and T-shirt had to be cut off. He was not shivering. David stated that Jason had stopped shaking just prior to the arrival of the police. Jason was tall, 5'8" (170 cm), and weighed no more than 130 lbs. (60 kg).

Jason's vital signs indicated continued unresponsiveness, a carotid pulse of 52 weak but regular, respirations now 6 and shallow, blood pressure neither audible nor palpable. Ventilations were assisted to increase his respiratory rate to 12 per minute. The ECG revealed a sinus bradycardia without ectopy. Warmed blankets were placed over his torso (thighs, abdomen, and chest), while his arms and lower legs were left exposed. Without IV access, nothing further could be accomplished at the scene, so Jason was quickly transported to the closest emergency room.

David's feet were carefully dried, with dressings placed between toes, and then wrapped in warm blankets. David said they had not consumed any alcohol and had not been smoking. He continued to experience uncontrollable shivering and his feet were starting to tingle as though tiny needles were pricking him. He was placed on warmed and humidified oxygen and had an IV inserted with normal saline. Though he was cold, his vital signs were normal and he was transported uneventfully to the hospital.

On arrival at the hospital, Jason's level of consciousness had not altered. His pulse had risen to 64 while his respirations remained at 6 per minute regular and shallow. Skin condition remained cold and pale, with lips cyanotic. Pupils continued to be dilated but reactive. Since the incident had taken place along the river shore in an outlying suburb of the city, the trip to hospital had taken approximately twenty minutes.

Multiple-Choice Questions

1. Heat loss is generated through which of the following?
1. conduction
2. convection
3. respiration
4. evaporation
5. radiation
    a) 1, 2, 4
    b) 1, 3, 5
    c) 1, 2, 4, 5
    d) 2, 3, 4, 5
    e) all of the above

2. Hypothermia is generally defined as a core body temperature of less than:
a) 96.8°F (36°C)
b) 95.0°F (35°C)
c) 93.2°F (34°C)
d) 91.4°F (33°C)
e) 89.5°F (32°C)

3. Individuals who are more susceptible to cold stress include the:

1. elderly
2. malnourished
3. chronically ill
4. very young

    a) 1, 2, 3
    b) 1, 3, 4
    c) 1, 2, 4
    d) 2, 3, 4
    e) all of the above

4. Disease states that diminish the capacity for heat production include:

1. cholecystitis
2. hypothyroidism
3. hypopituitarism
4. Parkinson's disease

    a) 1, 2
    b) 2, 3
    c) 2, 3, 4
    d) 1, 3, 4
    e) all of the above

5. During cold water immersion, heat loss may increase as much as:

    a) 5 times
    b) 10 times
    c) 15 times
    d) 20 times
    e) 25 times

6. The surface area of the head represents only 10 percent of the total body, yet heat loss may approximate:

    a) 5 to 10 percent
    b) 10 to 20 percent
    c) 20 to 30 percent
    d) 30 to 40 percent
    e) 40 to 50 percent

7. The clinical presentation of mild to moderate hypothermia generally includes:

1. amnesia
2. dyspnea
3. uncontrolled shivering
4. paradoxical undressing
5. ataxic gait
6. dysarthria
7. constricted pupils
8. lethargy and apathy

    a) 1, 2, 3, 5, 7
    b) 1, 3, 4, 7, 8
    c) 1, 3, 4, 5, 6, 8
    d) 2, 4, 5, 6, 7, 8
    e) all of the above

8. The clinical presentation of severe hypothermia often includes:

1. tachycardia
2. hypotension
3. lack of shivering
4. muscular rigidity
5. nausea and vomiting
6. hyperventilation
7. dysrhythmias
8. diaphoresis

    a) 2, 3, 4, 6, 7
    b) 1, 2, 3, 6, 8
    c) 1, 3, 4, 5, 7
    d) 2, 4, 5, 6, 7, 8
    e) all of the above

9. Complications arising from rewarming include the "after drop phenomenon" and "rewarming shock," which are associated with:

1. sending acidotic blood from the periphery back to the central circulation
2. sending warm blood by transfusion to the heart, causing arrhythmias
3. vigorous stimulation of victim causing ventricular fibrillation
4. a continued decline in core body temperature as warming is initiated

    a) 3
    b) 1, 4
    c) 2, 3
    d) 1, 3, 4
    e) all of the above

10. Passive and active external rewarming include warmed:
1. blankets
2. intravenous solutions
3. humidified oxygen
4. ambient environment

   a) 1, 4
   b) 1, 3
   c) 2, 3, 4
   d) 1, 2, 4
   e) all of the above

11. Frostbite pathology is associated with:
1. peripheral vasodilation
2. peripheral vasoconstriction
3. intracellular ice crystallization
4. interstitial ice crystallization

   a) 1
   b) 1, 4
   c) 2, 3
   d) 1, 3, 4
   e) 2, 3, 4

12. Which of the following statements referring to frostbite are accurate?
1. Fingers, hands, feet, toes, ears and nose are most commonly affected.
2. Immediate thawing is essential even if there is a risk of refreezing.
3. With stagnation of blood, ischemia will lead to necrosis, which can in turn lead to gangrene.
4. Severe deep frostbite is usually very painful and often described as a burning sensation.

   a) 1, 4
   b) 2, 3
   c) 1, 3
   d) 1, 2, 4
   e) 2, 3, 4

Debriefing

Living in a climate that exposes the population to sub-zero temperatures or more on a regular basis during the winter months means that many will be at risk for hypothermia. There are many definitions of accidental hypothermia, ranging from the simple "lowered body temperature" to the complex "unintentional decrease in the body's core temperature in the absence of preoptic anterior hypothalamic pathologic conditions." The latter is certainly a mouthful, but simply refers to a cooling of the body not related to a disease process affecting the thermoregulation center located in the hypothalamus.

Persons most at risk for accidental hypothermia include the very young, the elderly, the very thin, the mentally deficient, those suffering from dementia, alcohol and drug abusers, and the homeless. Lying in a snow bank is not the only source of exposure to a cold environment. Some elderly people who live alone on fixed incomes may, to reduce the high cost of heating, turn their thermostat down and thereby risk hypothermia, even while staying indoors.

The present scenario centers on exposure to an extremely cold environment. Two young teenagers develop accidental hypothermia, through cold-water immersion and subsequent exposure to sub-zero temperatures. Heat lost through direct contact with water is the result of conduction and produces a very rapid heat loss. Once out of the water, air currents passing over the body result in continued heat loss in the form of convection. Evaporation of water from soaked clothes on the body further increases the amount of heat lost, making it inevitable that hypothermia will develop quickly.

The body does attempt to compensate in the early stages, by vasoconstriction of peripheral blood vessels and shunting of blood to the core circulation. In this way, less blood is allowed to be cooled in outside tissues. Shivering initiates thermogenesis since the muscular activity increases the basal metabolic rate (BMR). A further increase in BMR is brought about through the release of the hormones adrenaline, thyroxin, and cortisol.

However, once the core body temperature falls below 32°C (89.5°F), these compensatory mechanisms begin to fail. Shivering stops at this stage, and if the body cools just a couple of degrees more, then even insulin is no longer fully effective in providing the cells with glucose essential to producing energy.

Since cooling is based on conduction, convection, and evaporation, a body will cool more rapidly if its surface area is increased proportional to its weight. That is, individuals who are tall and thin, having large surface areas, are at greater risk for rapid cooling than someone who is short and stocky. In this instance, Jason's total time of exposure was no more than 70 minutes overall, but it was plenty of time, given the factors involved (immersion in freezing water, sub-zero air temperature, wind-chill factor, and being relatively tall and thin) to create a situation of severe hypothermia.

Often forgotten in the overall picture of exposure is the wind-chill factor. A simplified calculation is to divide the wind speed in two, convert the result to a negative, and add the number to the temperature value. For wind chill to take effect there has to be an exposed heat source. Trees, for example, don't experience wind chill, but human beings, particularly with any exposed skin, will be at high risk. In cold environments, finding shelter from the wind can significantly increase the chance of survival.

An additional element, which was not encountered in this scenario but which could contribute to rapid cooling, is the consumption of alcohol. Alcohol vasodilates peripheral blood vessels, pooling warm blood in surface tissues;

this increases heat loss through radiation as a greater volume of blood is exposed to the cold. Alcohol is also a CNS depressant and can impair judgment, resulting in poor decision making.

Nicotine and caffeine are peripheral vasoconstrictors. While they do not contribute to generalized hypothermia, they can lead to frostbite, as circulation is restricted in the hands and feet. Fortunately, Jason and David had not contributed to their problems by smoking or drinking prior to their exposure.

With respect to treatment, the extent of Jason's hypothermia meant that he had to be treated gently. There is an anecdote about shipwrecked sailors who were subjected to exposure in life rafts. When rescued, they were required to climb ladders to board ship. This activity sent cold acidotic blood, which had pooled in skin and muscle tissues, back to the heart causing cardiac fibrillation. Many collapsed and died as they climbed aboard.

It is therefore important to take wet clothes off any severely hypothermic patient with a minimum of struggling and to cut them off when necessary. Insertion of endotracheal tubes is contraindicated since a vasovagal response could result in ventricular fibrillation. There is some evidence that an oropharyngeal airway should also be dispensed with, if a good airway can be maintained without it.

In hypothermia, although oxygen consumption decreases as core body temperature falls and basal metabolic rate slows, respiratory rates of 8 per minute that are extremely shallow may not be adequate, and ventilation of the patient should be assisted. Hyperventilation, however, could result in ventricular fibrillation and must be avoided.

It is easy to criticize the boys' actions—their lack of concern for their personal safety by walking on melting ice, and the poor decision on Jason's part not to go and get help but to stay with his friend, when staying meant having to immerse himself in freezing water—but in the end it serves little purpose. The number-one killer among teenage boys is trauma related accidents. Taking risks and poor judgment are part of a youthful belief in one's own immortality. It is hoped, however, that the lesson learned by experience will not come with a price too high to pay.

Follow-Up

David was treated for frostbite. His feet were rewarmed, by placing them in a warm bath with water temperature at 104°F (40°C). As the rewarming process continued, the feet became quite painful and analgesics were required. Eventually, David regained full sensation and use of his feet and toes.

Jason required internal rewarming for severe systemic hypothermia. A special thermometer capable of determining subnormal temperatures registered his core body temperature at 84.2°F (29°C). A warmed IV solution of D_5NS was introduced. Respiratory rate and depth improved while warmed humidified oxygen was continued. Pre-heated blankets were placed on the thorax and cardiac monitoring indicated normal sinus rhythm rate 68.

Peritoneal dialysis delivering dialysate heated to 107.6°F (42°C) was also introduced, as well as warm peritoneal lavage and warm gastric lavage.

Jason was admitted and continued to be monitored for cardiac dysrhythmia, and the development of cerebral edema. Rewarming proceeded at steady pace of a few degrees per hour, which resulted in a very positive outcome. Jason regained consciousness and suffered no neurological dysfunction.

Fact from Fiction

Marked cooling of body temperature produces profound vasoconstriction leading to blood stasis and coagulation. The poor perfusion that results leads to ischemic and necrotic tissue damage. In addition, ice crystals may form within cells causing many to rupture and die. As the microcirculation shuts down metabolic acidosis builds up.

Countering outside influences in temperature, internal thermogenesis results from the shivering and the release of epinephrine, cortisol, and thyroxine, which serve to increase the basal metabolic rate (BMR). As a consequence heat is produced in the form of kilocalories. Thermoregulation takes place in the hypothalamus, which may not function properly at two stages in our lives, when we are very young and very old.

An elderly person with a broken hip who has been lying on a basement floor where the temperature was 64°F (18°C) can easily experience hypothermia if left without blankets for any length of time. Equally serious, infants, particularly premature babies, who toss off their blankets in their cribs can be at risk for hypothermia. Without the ability to shiver and increase their BMR because of reduced stores of brown fat, they can experience hypothermia at a room temperature of 68°F (20°C).

Answer Key & Rationale

1. e) Conduction is the transfer of heat from a warm object to a cold object through direct contact.

Convection is the heat loss that occurs when currents of cold air disrupt the layer of warm air surrounding a body.

Respiration results in heat loss as the warmed moist air within the lungs is exhaled.

Evaporation cools the body when perspiration dissipates in the surrounding atmosphere.

Radiation results in heat loss by the normal generation of energy in the form of adenosine triphosphate (ATP), which is reflected in the basal metabolic rate (BMR).

2. b) Normal core (central) body temperature taken rectally ranges from 98°F (36.5°C) to 99.5°F (37.5°C). Hypothermia, a decrease in the body's core temperature, is generally defined as a rectal temperature of less than 95°F (35°C).

It is interesting to note that the extremities can withstand temperatures as much as 20 to 30 degrees lower than the torso, which houses the vital organs. Homeostasis requires a central body temperature range, which is very limited.

3. e) The elderly, whose circulatory systems are compromised due to age, are at greater risk for hypothermia. Those who are malnourished will have a lower BMR and have less subcutaneous fat, which insulates against the cold. Also included in this category are those suffering from kwashiorkor (malnutrition disease in children characterized by severe protein deficiency), marasmus (starvation and emaciation in children), and anorexia nervosa.

Patients who are chronically ill (for example, with emphysema, cardiovascular disease, or diabetes), are more susceptible to cold stress.

The very young—particularly infants, who as yet do not have the ability to shiver (a process of thermogenesis) as well as children who are not adequately protected from the elements—are also at increased risk from exposure.

4. c) Hypothyroidism, hypopituitarism, hypoadrenalism, and hypoglycemia are all failures of the endocrine system that can lead to decreases in heat production.

Parkinson's disease, CNS trauma, drug abuse (including alcohol), CVA, cerebellar lesion, neoplasm, and hypothalamic dysfunction may all result in impaired thermoregulation.

Associated clinical states, which run the risk of hypothermia, include burns, psoriasis, sepsis, pancreatitis, uremia, and acute spinal cord transection.

Cholecystitis refers to inflammation of the gallbladder and is not normally associated with any risk of hypothermia.

5. e) Cold water immersion is perhaps the most rapid form of heat loss. With water temperatures near freezing, conduction may increase heat loss as much as 25 times. Interestingly, immersion in cold water is also a method of treating cases of severe hyperthermia (heat stroke). It is therefore very important to remove wet clothing in order to arrest the loss of heat once the victim is removed from the water.

6. e) A tremendous amount of heat is lost through the head. Heat loss of 50 percent or more has been recorded in studies relating to exposure. Note also that the head surface area with children represents a greater proportion of the total body, placing them at greater risk. Protecting the head from environmental cold stress may be the single most important factor in the prevention of hypothermia.

7. c) Signs and symptoms that reflect mild to moderate hypothermia relate to a core body temperature between 95°F and 89.5°F (35°C–32°C). The distinction is made because at temperatures below 89.5°F (32°C) the compensatory mechanisms for thermogenesis, which include shivering, start to fail.

   Amnesia, shivering, ataxia, dysarthria, lethargy, and apathy are commonly associated with exposure. Paradoxical undressing may occur as hypothalamic control of vasoconstriction is lost and vasodilation occurs with loss of heat to the periphery. The hypothermic individual, therefore, feels suddenly warm and begins to remove clothing.

   Other clinical features may include confusion and disorientation, pale cool skin, tachycardia, tachypnea, increased blood pressure and, of course, a feeling of freezing.

8. a) Below a core temperature of 89.5°F (32°C), decompensation takes over and may result in hypotension, cessation of shivering, muscular rigidity with an inability to move, hyperventilation, dysrhythmia including sinus bradycardia, atrial fibrillation, ventricular fibrillation, and finally asystole.

   Ventricular fibrillation is a significant threat with core temperatures of 82.5°F (28°C) and below. Ventricular fibrillation does not respond well to therapy in the profoundly hypothermic patient.

   Other clinical features may include pulmonary edema, dilated pupils possibly non-reactive if below 80.5°F (27°C), coma, and a level of consciousness unresponsive to painful stimuli. Patients in severe hypothermia may have a barely detectable pulse, respirations of 2 to 3 per minute, and inaudible heart sounds. As a result, a person may be mistaken for dead; however, survival has occurred with core body temperatures as low as 68°F (20°C) because of the markedly decreased oxygen requirements of hypothermic tissues.

9. d) Blood that has been stagnant in the peripheral circulation becomes acidotic and if the extremities are warmed before the trunk, this acidotic blood will return to the central circulation, reducing the pH and causing an acid-base imbalance. Vigorous movement of the patient could also cause cold acidotic blood to enter the central circulation prematurely, which could cause a further decrease in core body temperature and potentiate ventricular fibrillation. This is known as the "after drop phenomenon."

   Rewarming shock refers to the process of vasodilation, which results as warming progresses. The subsequent relative hypovolemia, a reduced fluid volume (the result of cold diuresis) and a depletion of catecholamines (the result of prolonged shivering) means that the body is unable to maintain an adequate blood pressure.

Extreme cases of hypothermia may be treated with transfusions, as well as warm blood in a pump oxygenator circuit.

10. a) External rewarming refers to blankets, hot water bottles, heating pads, removal of wet clothing, isometric exercises to increase heat, and the provision of a warm environment, which could include warm baths.

Internal rewarming could include warm liquids if the patient is conscious, warmed intravenous solutions, warmed gastric and peritoneal lavage, as well as the inhalation of warmed oxygen.

11. e) As vasoconstriction of peripheral blood vessels occurs in order to maintain warmth in the central circulation, the perfusion of tissues in the extremities decreases. As freezing continues, water in both intra- and extracellular tissues forms ice crystals, which disrupt the cellular integrity of the membranes. The destruction of cell membranes along with ischemia leading to necrosis is the pathology, which results in frostbite.

12. c) The most commonly affected areas of frostbite are the extremities, where very little subcutaneous fat is able to protect against the elements. The fingers, hands, feet, toes, ears and nose are the first to succumb to frostbite. Left to continue freezing, deep third- and fourth-degree frostbite may occur resulting in necrosis which may result in gangrene over a period of days.

Rapid freezing, thawing, and refreezing are most damaging to tissues and if there is a substantial risk of refreezing, treatment should be delayed until the appropriate care can be provided.

Severe deep frostbite much like full-thickness burns is painless.

The initial symptoms of frostbite include numbness and paresthesia (often described as tingling) which progresses to anesthesia as nerve endings and pain receptors become frozen. Unfortunately, this may prevent the patient from recognizing the danger of irreversible tissue damage that occurs with continued exposure to cold.

CASE STUDY 5

911 RESPONSE: weakness and lethargy in an elderly female

The time was 6:50 A.M., ten minutes before the end of shift. The call coming through 911 and given out by dispatch indicated a possible cerebrovascular accident (CVA). An elderly female was unable to be awakened.

The building was a seniors' residence and the ambulance crew found their way to 1109 (the last door to the left down the corridor of the eleventh floor). They were greeted by an elderly gentleman, Mr. Bathgate, who appeared quite distraught. His distressed appearance was enhanced by the fact that he was in the early stages of Parkinson's disease and was exhibiting mild tremors in his hands. He directed the EMTs to the bathroom, where his wife, whose eyes were open, had been unable to talk or get up from the floor.

A quick overview of the scene revealed no obvious trauma. A neurological assessment was conducted once it was established that she had a radial pulse and respirations were adequate. The husband said that her name was Eleanor, and when he spoke her name, she seemed to show some slight recognition with incomprehensible words. The paramedics explained to Mrs. Bathgate who they were, that they were called by her husband who was concerned for her, and they were there to help.

Mrs. Bathgate was sitting on the bathroom floor leaning very much to her right. Grip strength was nonexistent in her right hand but was fairly strong in her left. This ability to follow instructions (to grip) indicated that she could understand verbal messages.

There were no signs of external head injuries, no bleeding on the scalp, no evidence of rhinorrhea or otorrhea, and no mastoid bruising. Pupils were equal and reactive. Consensual light reflexes were also present. Ptosis was evident along with an obvious drooping of the face, and a corner of her mouth was turned down.

Despite Mrs. Bathgate's ability to understand simple commands, she seemed quite confused. She was unable to point with her good (left) hand to the right day of the week when given the choice between three days written down on paper.

Information from her husband revealed a history of heart ailment for which she was taking digitalis. The medications were collected by the non-attending paramedic and placed in a bag to be brought to the hospital. The husband also divulged that his wife had experienced a number of fainting spells over the past couple of weeks. She had not sought medical attention, but had a doctor's appointment scheduled for later in the week.

Vital signs revealed a pulse of 68 strong and regular, respirations 16 regular and shallow, blood pressure 136/88, color good, and although the skin was warm and dry, there was poor skin turgor and she seemed dehydrated. The ECG indicated atrial fibrillation. A small but noticeable improvement in her mental status seemed to be taking place in that she would look more directly at the person speaking to her.

The paramedics reassured Mrs. Bathgate and explained how they were going to proceed. She was given a high concentration of oxygen and positioned right side down on the stretcher with the head of the stretcher slightly elevated. An IV was inserted with normal saline.

The paramedics proceeded to the hospital on the assumption that Mrs. Bathgate was probably suffering from a left-sided (L) cerebrovascular accident (CVA). En route a second set of vital signs revealed little change except that Eleanor's confusion and lack of communication seemed to be improving. She was able to talk and make some sense, although her words came slowly and were slurred.

Multiple-Choice Questions

1. Which of the following can lead to occlusive strokes?
1. aneurysms
2. arteriosclerosis
3. embolism
4. tumor

   a) 1, 2
   b) 3, 4
   c) 1, 3
   d) 2, 3, 4
   e) 1, 2, 4

2. In distinguishing between occlusive and hemorrhagic strokes, which of the following statements are true?
1. Occlusive strokes often occur in older people while they are asleep.
2. Hemorrhage strokes can occur in young people who seemed to be in excellent health prior to onset.
3. An intense headache is often a distinguishing feature of hemorrhagic strokes.

4. Hypertension is always a clue to the presence of occlusive strokes.
   a) 1, 2, 3
   b) 1, 3, 4
   c) 1, 2, 4
   d) 2, 3, 4
   e) all of the above

3. Patients at risk of cerebrovascular accidents are often those whose history includes:
   1. diabetes
   2. epilepsy
   3. hypertension
   4. heart disease
      a) 1, 2, 3
      b) 1, 3, 4
      c) 2, 3, 4
      d) 1, 2, 4
      e) all of the above

4. Patients at risk of cerebrovascular accidents are often those whose history includes:
   1. high cholesterol level
   2. use of oral contraceptives
   3. type A personality
   4. smoking
      a) 1, 3
      b) 1, 4
      c) 1, 2, 3
      d) 2, 3, 4
      e) 1, 2, 4

5. In differentiating between a right- and left-sided stroke which of the following are true?
   1. Left-sided strokes often affect the speech centers.
   2. Left-sided strokes often result in paralysis to the left side of the body.
   3. Right-sided strokes often result in hemiparesis contralaterally.
   4. Right-sided strokes often result in inappropriate affect, excessive laughing or crying.
      a) 1, 3
      b) 2, 4
      c) 2, 3
      d) 1, 2, 4
      e) 1, 3, 4

6. Which of the following statements are true of transient ischemic attacks (TIAs)?

1. Duration is usually minutes to an hour, but always less than twenty-four hours.
2. Signs and symptoms are usually the same as in a stroke.
3. Residual cerebral damage often leaves some paresis.
4. They may be a predictor of an eventual full-blown stroke.

   a) 1, 4
   b) 2, 4
   c) 1, 2, 4
   d) 1, 3, 4
   e) all of the above

7. Management of a patient with a stroke includes:

1. administration of a high concentration of oxygen
2. elevation of the patient's head twenty to thirty degrees
3. monitoring for cardiac dysrhythmia
4. being careful not to waste time explaining procedures; if the patient cannot speak, he/she probably cannot understand

   a) 1, 2
   b) 1, 3
   c) 2, 4
   d) 1, 3, 4
   e) 1, 2, 3

8. Hemorrhagic strokes commonly include the following etiology:

1. They often occur during stress or exertion.
2. They often are caused by a ruptured aneurysm arising at an arterial bifurcation.
3. Bleeding often occurs into the subarachnoid space.
4. Chronic systemic hypertension may result in intracerebral hemorrhage.

   a) 2, 4
   b) 3, 4
   c) 1, 2, 3
   d) 1, 2, 4
   e) all of the above

9. Cardinal signs of a subarachnoid bleed include:

1. Babinski reflex
2. nuchal rigidity
3. excruciating headache
4. vomiting

a) 1, 2, 3
b) 1, 3, 4
c) 2, 3, 4
d) 1, 2, 4
e) all of the above

10. Specific deficits seen in patients with strokes are related to the area of brain involved. Determine which of the following is/are true:

1. Posterior (vertebrobasilar) strokes are characterized by vertigo and ataxia.
2. Anterior cerebral artery strokes are characterized by amnesia and personality changes.
3. Middle cerebral artery strokes are characterized by dysphasia and contralateral hemiparesis.

    a) 3
    b) 1, 3
    c) 2, 3
    d) 1, 2
    e) 1, 2, 3

11. Transient ischemic attacks often involve:

1. vascular hemorrhage of small arterioles in the cerebrum
2. vascular occlusion usually caused by micro thrombi originating in major arteries or in the heart
3. platelet, fibrin, or other embolic material that lodges in a cerebral vessel and interferes transiently with blood flow
4. transient monocular blindness as a distinctive sign

    a) 1, 2, 3
    b) 2, 3, 4
    c) 1, 3, 4
    d) 1, 2, 4
    e) all of the above

12. Signs and symptoms commonly seen in patients with strokes are also associated with:

1. postictal (Todd's) paralysis
2. Bell's palsy
3. brain abscess
4. hyperglycemia

    a) 3, 4
    b) 1, 4
    c) 2, 3, 4
    d) 1, 2, 3
    e) all of the above

Debriefing

Many CVAs are called in just as people are waking up. The occlusive stroke, which most often occurs in older people, frequently comes on while they are asleep. In the morning, the spouse recognizes that something is wrong and calls for emergency help.

In this case, Mrs. Bathgate suffered her episode just after waking up, while in the bathroom. It is interesting to note that straining produces a Valsalva effect such that vasoconstriction of cerebral blood vessels reduces the diameter of arterioles and increases blood pressure. This may or may not have contributed in this case, since it is unclear as to whether Mrs. Bathgate had just entered or was just finishing in the bathroom.

The bathroom is often a very cramped space within which to work; however, it is necessary to assess for trauma before moving the patient. She could have had a spontaneous hip fracture or a syncopal episode and fallen, perhaps hitting her head on the enamel sink or bathtub. Even if the patient was in bed, she could have risen from the bed, suffered a spontaneous hip fracture, hit her head on a corner of the dresser and subsequently her husband may have helped her back in bed. Many calls given out as purely medical in nature often turn out to be trauma related. Therefore, assessment should consider possible traumatic injuries in even the most innocent of circumstances.

In this situation there were no obvious signs of traumatic injury, and the patient did not appear to be in shock. The fact that Mrs. Bathgate had a radial pulse that could easily be felt meant that her blood pressure was at least 80 systolic.

On the Glasgow Coma Scale, incomprehensive words or unintelligible noises ranks fairly low in the "best verbal response" category. However, she could control "eye opening" on command, and in the area of "motor response," she was able to follow commands, testing paresis through grip strength.

Since weakness was evidenced on the right side, it is possible that the lesion was located in the left hemisphere. Communication, including understanding and speech, are located in the left side of the brain in most people. Her verbal inadequacies may have been related to an affected area in her frontal lobe (Broca's area), usually in the left hemisphere, resulting in expressive aphasia. While her ability to communicate was hampered, she may still have been able to understand. For this reason it was essential for the paramedics to take the time to explain to Mrs. Bathgate who they were and why they were there, and to give an ongoing explanation of all procedures relating to assessment and treatment. Sometimes it helps to write down explanations, directions, or even answers for the patient. If these written messages are clear and simple, they may help to clarify the situation for the patient. They may also help to determine the patient's LOC more accurately.

Patients with a history of heart disease, particularly if it involves turbulent blood flow in the heart (as in the case of atrial fibrillation or valvular defects), are prone to the creation of emboli, which can find their way into cerebral blood vessels. Looking for antiarrhythmics or digitalis at the bedside table can therefore be of great help. It is also prudent to place all patients with a history of cardiac disease on the heart monitor. Remember: strokes are the third leading cause of death behind heart disease and cancer.

There are two clues that suggest that Mrs. Bathgate suffered from a transient ischemic attack (TIA) as opposed to a full stroke. Mr. Bathgate provided the first clue when he told the EMTs that his wife had experienced similar episodes of syncope over the past couple of weeks. The second clue reflects the transient nature of TIAs: Mrs. Bathgate's incomprehensible speech began to dissipate en route, so that she was making herself understood. The full extent of her recovery would determine whether it was indeed a TIA or a CVA.

The vital signs were unremarkable for the most part. Blood pressure tends to rise as people get older, so the initial BP of 136/88 should be noted more for the pulse pressure of 48 and used as a base line for the second set. Cerebral edema will often accompany an occlusive stroke with an increase in intracranial pressure dependent on the extent of damage.

Mrs. Bathgate was possibly suffering from dehydration, which, when combined with other risk factors, can precipitate strokes.

Depending on time available, the EMTs could have performed a more complete neurological assessment including the twelve cranial nerves. This is particularly important when dealing with TIAs, since the effects may be seen only for a short time (they usually resolve in under one hour), and the area of involvement as determined by the neuro assessment can be very helpful to the hospital staff. Over a third of all CVAs are preceded by TIAs, so early diagnosis and treatment may help prevent the devastation of a full-blown stroke.

In managing the stroke patient, delivering a high concentration of oxygen is important since the brain is very susceptible to hypoxia. Head elevation promotes cerebral venous drainage, offsetting cerebral edema. If the stroke is extensive or hemorrhagic in origin and the respiratory rate drops, then hyperventilation is required both to improve oxygenation and to decrease intracranial pressure.

Mrs. Bathgate was placed on her affected side in order to allow her independence of movement with her least-affected arm free. By placing her on her side, the EMTs could properly monitor her airway. Needless to say, a stroke is a frightening event to all concerned and empathetic reassurance is important to both the patient and the spouse.

Follow-Up

Mrs. Bathgate recovered fully in the hospital over a short period of two hours and was diagnosed with a TIA. Her current list of medications was evaluated, and it was discovered that she had discontinued taking an anticoagulant (Coumadin) because she had run out of it. She was placed on enteric (coated) aspirin therapy.

Fact from Fiction

There has been more than a 50 percent decline in stroke mortality over the past quarter century. Since the incidence of stroke has remained unchanged, the number of patients requiring long-term care and rehabilitation has risen greatly and makes strokes the leading cause of serious disability.

Among the survivors, almost half have some form of hemiparesis; many are unable to walk. A significant number remain aphasic and almost a third of all stroke victims are clinically depressed. More than half are no longer able to independently perform activities of daily living.

A transient ischemic attack is an event where associated neurological deficits completely resolve. If the event is an embolus(i)/thrombus(i) and not the result of vasospasm then the clot(s) is/are efficiently lysed by the endogenous fibrinolytic system before permanent tissue damage occurs. Of note, however, is that one or more TIA episode increases the risk of stroke by about tenfold. An acute ischemic stroke produces irreversable cellular damage (necrosis) within several minutes, however, surrounding the infarct is a larger area of ischemic yet viable cells called the "penumbra." The goal of early intervention with thrombolytic therapy is to salvage the penumbra. To have maximal effect and prevent further brain damage definitive treatment should be initiated within three hours of the event, hence the saying "time is brain."

When referring to a stroke the term "brain attack" has been popularized to educate the public about the importance of seeking care early. This is in keeping with the successful campaign to educate the public on the risk factors and early warning signs of a "heart attack." In addition to educating the public, the term "brain attack" has been coined to shake the established medical community out of its historic rut concerning stroke. In the past, the attitude about CVA was that it was an event that was over before anyone could do anything and, because brain damage is permanent damage, there was little that could be done for the patient. Therefore, there was no need to rush.

Recent research, however, has pointed out that CVA is an ongoing event and the ultimate outcome for the patient can be significantly reduced by reducing time to definitive treatment. Time means brain tissue and the quicker that care can be provided, the less damage is done. Today, some of the most promising work on emergency treatment of stroke victims has to do with the use of thrombolytic drugs. In much the same way that thrombolytics reduce the severity of heart attacks by dissolving clots and reperfusing ischemic heart tissue, the same drugs seem to work in the same way with CVA. Quickly reperfusing brain tissue may reduce or eliminate long-term damage. These are patients for whom time makes a huge difference in their outcome.

Answer Key & Rationale

1. d) Occlusive strokes take different forms: arteriosclerosis resulting in a reduction in the diameter of the arterial wall; embolism in the form of a thrombosis, fat, amniotic fluid, or air; or a tumor resulting in exterior pressure on an artery. A cerebral aneurysm (weakened area of a blood vessel), once ruptured, would result in bleeding into the brain and is defined as a hemorrhagic stroke.

2. a) Since precipitating factors such as arteriosclerosis and heart disease often take years to develop, occlusive strokes are most often seen among the elderly. The highest incidence is among those between 75 and 85 years of age. These strokes often occur during sleep.

   Hemorrhagic strokes often occur as a result of a congenital aneurysm and can strike with little advanced noticed. There is often an excruciating headache associated with this type of stroke.

   Hypertension may be found in the history of both types of strokes, with a slightly higher incidence found among those with hemorrhagic strokes.

3. b); **4.** e) Risk factors for the development of cerebrovascular accidents include heart disease in particular arrhythmias and valvular defects, as well as arteriosclerosis. Arteriosclerosis itself has the following risk factors: hypertension, smoking, elevated blood cholesterol, diabetes mellitus, and sedentary lifestyle.

   Other risk factors of CVA include the use of oral contraceptives, coagulation disorders, chronic hypoxia, and hypothyroidism.

5. e) The temporal lobe in the dominant hemisphere of the brain controls the speech center and can often be affected with a left-sided CVA. Since the corticospinal tracts cross just below the brainstem, a CVA in the right hemisphere may result in weakness to the left side of the patient. A left-sided CVA consequently results in paresis to the right side of the patient.

   While it is difficult to generalize, right-sided CVAs often involve a personality change that results in impatience and increased lability.

6. c) TIAs usually last only a few minutes, rarely more than eight hours and always less than twenty-four hours. The deficits manifested often resolve within fifteen minutes to an hour. The physical findings are the same as those of a stroke; however, after resolution findings are unremarkable. Patients with new episodes, or increasing frequency of TIAs, are at risk of a full blown stroke.

7. e) Management for a stroke patient includes a high concentration (12 to 15 lpm) of oxygen since the brain is particularly sensitive to hypoxia. Head elevation promotes venous drainage and minimizes cerebral edema. Cardiac monitoring is a good precaution against further complications and is of particular importance for those patients with a history of heart disease. Always explain procedures and provide reassurance to patients. Many patients who are unable to communicate can nonetheless hear and understand what is taking place around them.

8. e) Pressure on arterial walls increases during times of stress and exertion, and may in turn result in the rupture of an existing aneurysm. The most common location of cerebral aneurysms is at an arterial bifurcation along the circle of Willis, with bleeding into the subarachnoid space. Uncontrolled, prolonged hypertension can also result in the rupture of small arterioles deep within the brain.

9. c) The three most common signs of a subarachnoid bleed are nuchal rigidity, a very intense (sometimes described as excruciating) headache, and vomiting (often projectile).

The Babinski reflex, if found to exist, may be a sign of a stroke. However, it does not differentiate between an occlusive or hemorrhagic stroke.

10. e) Stroke victims experience problems directly related to the damaged area of the brain.

A cerebrovascular accident (CVA) involving the vertebral basilar system may show evidence of vertigo and ataxia, as well as dysmetria, dysphagia, dysarthria, diplopia, nystagmus, tinnitus, and hearing loss.

A CVA involving the anterior cerebral artery may result in amnesia and personality changes (flat affect or apathy as examples), as well as confusion, preservation, incontinence, contralateral hemiparesis or hemiplegia, apraxia, and expressive aphasia (for dominant hemisphere involvement).

A CVA involving the middle cerebral artery may result in dysphasia and contralateral hemiparesis, as well as a denial or lack of recognition of a paralyzed extremity, hemianopia, and an inability to turn the eyes toward the affected side.

11. b) TIAs represent thrombotic particles made up of platelets and fibrin, which cause an intermittent blockage of cerebral circulation. Thrombi may form wherever there is turbulent blood flow, which often arises where plaques form on artery walls, or with atrial or valvular dysfunction in the heart. Transient monocular blindness (amaurosis fugax) is often a presenting sign of TIA.

Since a TIA represents temporary disruption in cerebral blood flow, mostly of an occlusive nature, it is not representative of a hemorrhagic stroke.

12. d) Postictal (Todd's) paralysis, seen with epileptic seizures, represents a transient hemiparesis or hemiplegia which could be mistaken for a CVA or TIA.

Bell's palsy is a neuropathy of the facial nerve, resulting in paralysis of the muscles on one side of the face. There is usually sagging on one side of the mouth such that the patient may drool and be mistaken for a CVA.

A brain abscess may show all the signs of a stroke; however, there are some dissimilarities in history and clinical manifestation.

Hyperglycemia is not likely to present with stroke-like symptoms, but hypoglycemia may. Common similarities between CVAs and hypoglycemia include hemiparesis, confusion, facial drooping, and diplopia.

Not listed in the question, but also of significance: a CVA may be mistaken for alcohol intoxication, which depresses the CNS, producing stroke-like symptoms (confusion, dysarthria, and impaired gait, for example).

CASE STUDY 6

The call came just as the paramedics sat down to eat a very late lunch. Six hours of back-to-back calls and still no time for lunch. Since this was not unusual, it hardly received a grumble.

The call referred to a domestic problem, nature unknown, involving a male (forty) acting strangely. The police had been advised and were responding. The priority assigned by dispatch was urgent but not life threatening, so lights and siren were not engaged. The paramedics were counting on the police to arrive first and secure the scene. There is really no telling what dangers may present themselves in calls labeled "domestic disturbance" and the crew felt safer if the police officers made the initial contact.

As it happened, the family members were all sitting quietly in the living room with worried looks on their faces. Once the police established that violence had not been perpetrated, or even threatened, they stepped aside to allow the paramedics to investigate further. The call was instigated by the eleven-year-old son who was worried that his dad was not well. Other members of the family present included a nine-year-old boy and a six-year-old girl. The father, dressed in pajamas, was lying on the couch and appeared unaware of what was taking place around him.

The father, after repeated questioning, finally gave his name as Peter DiAngelo. Mr. DiAngelo appeared confused and not well oriented to either place or time. Although the paramedics had initially introduced themselves, he seemed not to know who they were or why they were there. They introduced themselves a second time.

From the eldest son, whose name was Richard, it was established that Mr. DiAngelo was forty-four, a single parent, his wife having died of breast cancer three years ago. Richard said his dad got up that morning but did not dress or go to work. The children had gone to school and when they arrived home they found their dad on the couch swearing at them, something he had never done before. They were afraid something was wrong with him, so they called 911.

Further information revealed that Peter DiAngelo never missed a day of work even if he had a bad cold. He had been a construction worker for over twenty years, and to Richard's knowledge had no history of any illnesses, and he was not on any medication. There had been no complaints of recent infections, not even a toothache. Richard stated that his dad had been in the hospital after a fall on the construction site. X-rays had been taken because he had hit his head on some scaffolding, but he had come home the same day. Richard said that this incident occurred about two weeks ago, and all seemed okay until today.

The two younger children were also questioned and added that their dad had complained of headaches over the past couple of days.

Assessment revealed no evidence of trauma: no hematomas, no scalp lacerations, no mastoid bruising, no periorbital ecchymosis, no rhinorrhea, no otorrhea, no bleeding from nose or ears, no evidence of ptosis or facial palsies. No alcohol was detected on the breath. Although Mr. DiAngelo seemed increasingly somnolent, having to be roused to open his eyes, his speech was not slurred. Pupils were small at 3 mm, but equal and reactive to both consensual and direct light reflexes. Testing for ocular movement proved unremarkable and his vision seemed to be normal.

Respirations were rapid and deep while the pulse was 62 strong and regular. Blood pressure was 146/76, and skin condition was warm to touch with good color. The ECG showed a normal sinus rhythm without any abnormalities. A check of blood glucose revealed a normal level of 95. When questioned, he seemed confused; questions often had to be repeated a number of times before a response was forthcoming. Even then his sentences had a tendency to trail off without being completed. Nonetheless, the crew determined that he had no complaints, no headache presently, no nausea or vomiting, no evidence of nuchal rigidity. He expressed only a desire to be left alone in order to sleep.

The necessity for in-hospital assessment was explained to Mr. DiAngelo and he did not object as he received a high concentration of oxygen and preparations were made for transport. An IV was inserted with normal saline to keep the vein open for access if needed.

With deteriorating level of consciousness (LOC) as the chief complaint and a previous history of head trauma (despite the time interval since the accident), the patient was treated as a potential head injury/neurological illness. The head of the stretcher was elevated 30 degrees and he was positioned semi-prone in order to ensure an adequate airway in case vomiting occurred.

Before departure, while the attending paramedic took a second set of vital signs, the second paramedic explained to all three children that their dad would be well taken care of, that he was going to the hospital to find out why he wasn't feeling himself. The police were going to stay with the children while an aunt was called to come over.

The second set of vital signs revealed a slightly slower pulse rate of 54, still strong. Respirations were unchanged, rapid, and deep, while the blood pressure rose slightly to 154/76. Skin condition remained unchanged. The right pupil was now slightly larger than the left and Mr. DiAngelo reacted with mumbling and groans when the paramedics tried to arouse him.

The call priority was upgraded to an emergency, and a call to the hospital was conducted en route, listing neurological status and the most recent set of vital signs.

Multiple-Choice Questions

1. Damage to brain tissue can result from:
1. a direct blow
2. rapid deceleration
3. intracranial bleeding
4. herniation
5. cerebral edema

   a) 1, 2, 4
   b) 1, 3, 5
   c) 2, 3, 4, 5
   d) 1, 2, 3, 4
   e) all of the above

2. Which of the following statements refers to a concussion?
1. It often results in residual neurological deficit.
2. Loss of consciousness often is greater than five minutes.
3. Half of all concussions involve linear skull fractures.
4. It is generally defined as a transient loss of consciousness.

   a) 4
   b) 1, 2
   c) 2, 4
   d) 1, 3, 4
   e) 1, 2, 3

3. Statements that reflect the pathology of a contusion include:

1. Severity is related to the amount of energy transmitted to underlying brain tissue.
2. Effects on cerebral tissue include bleeding and edema resulting from bruising.
3. Hemorrhage and brain swelling are at their peak in the first one to two hours after injury.
4. Injury may result from coup, contrecoup, or shearing forces.

   a) 1, 2, 3
   b) 1, 3, 4
   c) 1, 2, 4
   d) 2, 3, 4
   e) all of the above

4. Which of the following statements referring to epidural hematomas are correct?

1. Bleeding most often results from hemorrhage of the middle meningeal artery.
2. The most common site of an extradural hematoma is over the occipital lobe.
3. The most common cause of epidural hemorrhage is motor vehicle accidents.
4. The age group most associated with this type of intracranial bleed is forty to sixty.

   a) 1, 3
   b) 2, 3
   c) 1, 2, 4
   d) 2, 3, 4
   e) all of the above

5. Subdural hematomas may be classified as:

1. acute
2. subacute
3. chronic
4. shaken baby syndrome

   a) 1, 2
   b) 1, 2, 3
   c) 2, 3, 4
   d) 1, 3, 4
   e) all of the above

6. The clinical course that best describes the elements common to both epidural and subdural hematomas is:

a) acute and progressive deterioration of neurological function leading to brainstem herniation

b) initially no loss of consciousness; then, as the lesion develops, increased intracranial pressure leads to coma

c) immediate loss of consciousness with rapid deterioration of neurological status resulting in conning

d) brief period of unconsciousness followed by lucidity of varying duration progressing to a decreasing LOC

e) amnesia surrounding the event leading to altered personality followed by depressed mental functioning

7. Clinical manifestations relating to intracranial hemorrhage may include:

1. ipsilateral pupil dilation
2. tachycardia
3. altered personality
4. skin cold, pale
5. ataxic respirations
6. projectile vomiting

    a) 2, 3, 4, 5
    b) 1, 3, 5, 6
    c) 1, 2, 4, 6
    d) 1, 3, 4, 5
    e) 1, 2, 3, 6

8. Clinical manifestations relating to intracranial hemorrhage may include:

1. ipsilateral hemiparesis
2. Cheyne-Stokes respirations
3. bilateral pupil constriction
4. increased temperature
5. increased pulse pressure
6. paradoxical pulse

    a) 1, 4, 5
    b) 3, 4, 6
    c) 1, 2, 3, 5
    d) 1, 2, 4, 6
    e) 2, 3, 4, 5

9. Clinical manifestations relating to intracranial hemorrhage may include:

1. confusion, disorientation
2. bradycardia
3. hypotension

4. hyperventilation
5. decorticate posturing
6. decerebrate posturing

    a) 1, 4, 5
    b) 1, 2, 3, 6
    c) 1, 2, 3, 4
    d) 1, 2, 4, 5, 6
    e) 2, 3, 4, 5, 6

10. Long-term effects of traumatic head injury can include:

1. chronic headaches
2. mental dysfunction
3. motor dysfunction
4. post-traumatic epilepsy

    a) 1, 2, 4
    b) 1, 3, 4
    c) 1, 2, 3
    d) 2, 3, 4
    e) all of the above

11. Patients most at risk of chronic subdural hematomas are:

1. elderly persons
2. alcoholics
3. patients on long-term anticoagulants
4. those with blood dyscrasia

    a) 1, 2, 3
    b) 1, 2, 4
    c) 2, 3, 4
    d) 1, 3, 4
    e) all of the above

12. Early management of intracranial bleeding includes:

1. Trendelenburg or shock positioning
2. hyperventilation to decrease intracranial pressure (ICP)
3. reducing external stimuli
4. providing spinal immobilization

    a) 2, 3, 4
    b) 1, 3, 4
    c) 1, 2, 3
    d) 1, 2, 4
    e) all of the above

Debriefing

Even though this was not a case of family violence, there was no way of knowing ahead of time whether or not police assistance would be necessary. It is always best to take a cautious approach. The dispatchers who receive incoming calls are given very limited and often contradictory information. They do an excellent job under the circumstances, considering that the information often comes from someone who is highly excited about what has just occurred, whose heightened anxiety level may be blocking important information, and who does not likely have medical training. Unfortunately, family disputes too often erupt in violence; police should be present whenever this possibility exists. The only appropriate protection for prehospital providers is to ensure, whenever possible, that police are first to enter any potentially dangerous scene.

In cases where the chief complaint is altered level of consciousness there is always an initial question as to whether the origin or etiology is more psychological or pathological in nature. It is not uncommon for EMTs to find an adult suffering from clinical depression, who has not dressed for the day, who is lethargically lying on the couch, who may have consumed alcohol or taken an overdose of pills. Mr. DiAngelo fits aspects of this picture; moreover, he has recently lost a close loved one. All possibilities require investigation, but there are also contradictions in this case. Depression is most often chronic, with a long history that reflects on both work and family. Mr. DiAngelo was not known to have been drinking; alcohol was not noticed on his breath; he apparently had never missed a day of work; and the children felt that he was so out of character they found it necessary to phone for help.

The most experienced paramedics have a sixth sense that would help them recognize that the clues in this situation do not quite add up to clinical depression. Not surprisingly, the most relevant questions asked are those by the senior paramedics. However, even rookies stand a good chance of shedding light on the situation if their approach is logical and methodical. In this case, evaluation of the chief complaint means an accurate assessment of the level of consciousness. In this respect it is important to clarify terminology. Unconsciousness is fairly clear to all, but the meaning of semi-consciousness falls into a grey area where a precise definition is difficult to pin down. Terms that are open to interpretation should be avoided.

Confusion refers to the loss of ability to think rapidly and clearly, and is also associated with impaired judgment and decision making. *Disorientation* initially involves failure to identify time followed by place, and finally it involves a loss of self-recognition which is the last to be lost. *Lethargy* results in limited spontaneous movement or speech, although the patient remains easily aroused to normal speech and touch; it may or may not involve orientation to person, place, and time. *Somnolence* or *obtundation* reveals mild to moderate reduction in arousal (awareness) with limited response to the environment; also, the patient falls asleep unless stimulated verbally or by touch, and responses to questions are at a minimum. *Stupor* is a condition of deep sleep from which a person may be aroused or caused to respond verbally or physically only by vigorous and repeated stimulation; response is often purposeful (grabbing) or withdrawal. *Coma* is a state of unresponsiveness to any noxious or painful stimuli.

A very useful tool in evaluating a patient's neurological status is the Glasgow Coma Scale (GCS). Originally intended as a prognostic indicator, it provides a clear recording system for stimulus and response. Most patient care reports have a section where the GCS is recorded.

The pupils play an important part in the evaluation of neurological status. In this case they were quite small, which raises two main concerns. First is the possibility of drugs on board; in particular, narcotics (morphine for example) will create pinpoint pupils. The overall effect of this family of drugs is to depress the central nervous system, which would be reflected in a slow and shallow respiratory rate. However, Mr. DiAngelo's rapid and deep respirations (setting aside a metabolic imbalance) seem to point away from a toxic element. A second possible cause of pinpoint pupils is pressure on the oculomotor nerve in the area of the midbrain. The potential for an ongoing lesion should lead to a further assessment of ocular movement and vision. The integrity of the fourth, sixth, and second cranial nerves may provide clues to the extent of an expanding mass.

The deterioration in Mr. DiAngelo's level of consciousness along with the changes in vital signs—decreasing heart rate, widening pulse pressure, unequal pupils (an ominous sign)—combine to indicate increasing intracranial pressure (ICP). This would tend to point in the direction of an expanding lesion, possibly intracerebral hemorrhage, ruptured aneurysm, subacute or chronic subdural hematoma; however, the existence of a brain tumor, abscess, encephalitis, or meningitis cannot be completely ruled out. The absence a couple of signs (such as fever and nuchal rigidity) may lessen the possibility of a particular disease process but in no way eliminates it. The task of the EMT is to gather as much relevant information as possible and provide patient management for what may be termed a general field diagnosis; however, the definitive diagnosis always remains with the hospital emergency staff. This statement, although obvious, should always be kept in mind when reporting assessment findings.

Children deserve special consideration and attention when they are involved in a primary care setting. First it was important in this case to acknowledge their concern about their dad and to reassure them that they did the best thing possible by calling for help. They had experienced a tremendously difficult situation with the loss of their mother and now with their father ill, they were extremely frightened and anxious. Including children in the information gathering may not only provide useful clues but will also give them a feeling that they are helping. Taking the time to listen to their concerns and honestly reassuring them will help them cope with situations like this one.

Follow-Up

Mr. DiAngelo, with the aid of computerized tomography (CT scan) and magnetic resonance imaging (MRI), was diagnosed as having a subacute subdural hematoma, most probably secondary to the earlier work-related head trauma. Increasing intracranial pressure was alleviated through surgical intervention. A mass (clot) the size of a golf ball located superior and frontal was evacuated without complications.

Mannitol, a hyperosmolar drug, was given to reduce cerebral edema by drawing excess water from the brain and reabsorbing it in the bloodstream. Dexamethasone (Decadron), an anti-inflammatory steroid that has little salt-retaining action, and furosemide (Lasix), a powerful diuretic, were also introduced. Antibiotics were given to reduce the risk of infection post-surgically.

Recovery for Peter DiAngelo progressed well with no permanent impairment of mental functioning, although a residual gaze palsy did persist for a short time. A large and close extended family was able to provide support for his children during his recovery, and he was able to return to work within a few weeks of being discharged from the hospital.

Fact from Fiction

Increased intracranial pressure (ICP) occurs when there is a rise in volume within the cranium. Except for neonates, the skull is a rigid closed system and contains approximately 80 percent brain tissue, 10 percent blood, and 10 percent cerebrospinal fluid (CSF). Normal pressure within the cranium ranges from 0 to 15 mmHg. A compensatory relationship exists where a change in volume in any of the three components can be offset by a reduction in the volume of the other two. By limiting blood flow to the head, displacing CSF (pulling water out of brain tissue into the blood and excreting it through the kidneys), the overall pressure buildup may be limited or reduced. The brain's ability to tolerate increases in volume without a corresponding increase in pressure is referred to as compliance.

When a head injury occurs the ICP will remain normal until the compensatory mechanisms reach their limit. Once this happens a negative cycle begins where the ongoing lesion, in shifting brain tissue, compromises blood flow to the brain. The hope is that a tamponade effect will limit the progress of the lesion, however, the result is often an increase in tissue ischemia leading to cerebral edema and a further increase in ICP. Since the highly specialized cortical neurons are very sensitive to oxygen deficit, a decrease in level of consciousness may be the most important clue to an early rise in ICP. Once pressure has risen to the point of forcing brainstem herniation it may well be too late.

Answer Key & Rationale

1. e) Injury to brain tissue can be the result of trauma, a direct blow that may or may not fracture the skull. Underlying damage results in contusion, intracranial hemorrhage, and edema. Deceleration injury results from indirect trauma called a coup and contracoup. In this situation, brain tissue violently confronts the inner ridges of the skull.

Types of intracranial bleeding include epidural and subdural hematoma, intracerebral and subarachnoid hemorrhage, as well as the bleeding that occurs with a basilar skull fracture. Herniation occurs as increased pressure in one compartment of the cranial vault pushes or shifts brain tissue to an area of lower pressure. Increased pressure on a particular area of the brain, through herniation, will compromise that area's blood supply, producing additional ischemia and hypoxia.

Cerebral edema occurs with damage to the capillaries following injury. The loss of vascular integrity results in increased capillary permeability. Edema may also occur in areas of ischemia and necrosis where the release of lysosomes from intracellular compartments result in an increase in the blood-brain barrier's permeability. Cerebral edema may develop over hours or over several days, increasing intracranial pressure and potentiating herniation.

2. a) A concussion is often poorly defined but the term generally indicates a transient loss of consciousness lasting no longer than five minutes and leaving no permanent or residual brain damage. Most concussions do not involve skull fractures. A skull fracture may be an indicator of underlying injury but it is not a measure of it. Rarely, the effects of a concussion may persist for weeks or months depending on the severity of the injury. A post-concussive syndrome can include headache, nervousness or anxiety, insomnia, depression, and fatigability.

3. c) A contusion represents a bruising of brain tissue, the size dependent on the force and energy transmitted from the initial trauma. The injury may stem from direct or indirect violence resulting in a coup, contracoup, or rotational injury from shearing forces. Bleeding and edema occur within the contused area and are at their peak twelve to twenty-four hours after injury. Recovery of consciousness may be slow and residual neurological deficits can persist for prolonged periods of time.

4. a) Epidural hematoma, also called extradural hematoma, is a collection of blood that results from bleeding between the dura matter and the skull. Eighty-five percent of epidural hematomas involve a tear in the middle meningeal artery, while 15 percent result from injury to the meningeal vein or dural sinus. The most common site of an epidural hematoma is over the temporal lobe because the meningeal artery runs in a groove on

the surface of the temporal bone. Less common sites of extradural hemorrhage include areas over the subfrontal and occipital-suboccipital lobes.

Motor vehicle accidents are the most common cause of epidural
hematomas, although injuries have also resulted from falls and sporting
accidents. As a consequence, the age group most commonly associated
with this injury includes people aged twenty to forty.

5. b) A subdural hematoma refers to a collection of blood, usually venous,
between the dura matter and the arachnoid membrane. Acute subdural
hematomas usually develop within hours and are most often located over
the top of the skull. Half are associated with skull fractures, with the most
common cause being motor vehicle accidents. Subacute subdural
hematomas develop more slowly, usually over a few days to a week or two.

The clinical presentation is the same for both acute and subacute subdural hematomas. Chronic subdural hematomas may take weeks to
develop and are most often seen among the elderly, alcoholics, persons
on long-term anticoagulant therapy, or those with blood dyscrasia.

Although not considered part of the classification for subdural
hematomas, when seen in infants it is often the result of physical child
abuse and has been termed by some "shaken baby syndrome."

6. d) Trauma leading to either epidural or subdural hemorrhage often follows
a pattern in which there is an initial loss of consciousness, followed by a
lucid period with often complete orientation. Then, after a period of time,
depending on the extent and nature of bleed either arterial or venous,
there follows a deterioration in neurological functioning. If the build up
in intracranial pressure (ICP) continues unabated, then 'conning' (the
descriptive term for herniation of the brain stem through the foramen
magnum) may result. Pressure on the pons and cerebellum will be manifested in altered respirations, pulse, and blood pressure, as well as decorticate and decerebrate posturing in the end stages.

7. b); **8.** e); **9.** d) Signs and symptoms associated with intracranial hemorrhage
include altered level of consciousness, which may present as confusion,
disorientation, personality changes such as combative or uncooperative
behavior, lethargy, somnolence, stupor, or coma. Motor dysfunction may
present as gait disturbances, contralateral hemiparesis or hemiplegia,
seizures, purposeful movement or withdrawal to painful stimuli, decorticate or decerebrate posturing, or total unresponsiveness. Vital signs may
be altered revealing: bradycardia; hypertension with widened pulse pressure; varying respiratory patterns such as Cheyne Stokes, Biot's, hyperventilation, ataxic, and apneustic; constricted or dilated ipsilateral or
bilateral pupils which may react, may be sluggish, or may be non-reactive; as well as elevated body temperature with skin warm and dry.
Vomiting, particularly projectile vomiting, is not uncommon.

It is interesting to note that the signs and symptoms of head injury
patients are often in opposition to those seen in shock. When presented

with trauma, if both tachycardia and hypotension are present, hemorrhage other than intracranial should be suspected.

10. e) In dealing with head injuries, a variety of neurological problems may be experienced long after the initial insult. Chronic headaches as well as mental and motor dysfunction are not uncommon. Organic brain damage, and post-traumatic epilepsy resulting from scar formation are also possible sequels to head injury.

11. e) Chronic subdural hematomas can develop over a period of weeks often as the result of minor trauma to individuals with a secondary pathology. Those most at risk include the elderly, alcoholics, persons with blood dyscrasia, and patients on long-term anticoagulants.

12. a) The proper positioning for the head-injury patient is head elevated approximately thirty degrees, allowing for venous drainage and decreasing the potential for ICP. Spinal immobilization should be the protocol for all victims of traumatic head injury. If cervical and spinal injury can be ruled out, then a semi-prone position would allow for proper airway maintenance, particularly since vomiting is a commonly associated symptom.

The delivery of a high oxygen concentration along with hyperventilation is probably the most effective method of reducing rising intracranial pressure in the field. Cerebral hypoxia leads to increased acidosis, which causes vasodilation of the cerebral vasculature, which in turn compromises the space available for brain tissue (remember: the brain is contained within the cranial vault with no room for expansion). Increased oxygenation and the blowing off of carbon dioxide will reduce the acidosis and help counteract rising pressure.

Reducing external stimuli such as keeping the noise level to a minimum (talking softly, restricting the use of the siren) will help prevent any rapid increase in intracranial pressure.

CASE STUDY 7

The call was outside the city, not far out, but still the driving was slow. Even though it was 3:30 in the morning and the highway was deserted, fog slowed the medic unit's progress. Fog had settled in thick and dense, making visibility a problem. The house, a Cape Cod-style bungalow, was on County Road 8, four miles down from the intersection with the highway. Even reading road signs was difficult.

There was very little information coming through dispatch: an expectant mother with a severe headache. The houses were set back from the road, making them difficult to see. The ambulance crew, not surprisingly, overshot the address and radioed to have someone from the house in question turn on the four-way flashers on a car in their driveway. The Paramedics subsequently found their way to the flashing car. The house, barely visible, was painted a blue gray, which blended in well with the fog.

A fourteen-year-old boy met the crew at the door and said that his stepmother was now complaining of stomach cramps and "might be having the baby." His father was out of town on business and was not expected back for two days. The paramedics, while being led to the bedroom, thanked him for turning on the lights to the car.

Janice Forest was thirty-six-years-old and experiencing her first pregnancy. She was lying fully dressed in bed with her knees drawn up. She was in her thirty-fourth week with twins and everything seemed to be going well up to now. Her latest ultrasound indicated that all was proceeding normally.

She complained of a headache with blurred vision as well as epigastric abdominal pain that was diffuse and steady.

When asked, Janice stated that she had been getting headaches over the past few days and felt that she was putting on a little more weight than normal. Her hands and feet were a little swollen and causing her discomfort, particularly on her ring finger.

There had been no bleeding, her water had not yet broken, and the abdominal pain was steady, rather than coming at intervals. She had last seen her obstetrician three weeks ago without complaints and was not on any prescribed medication. Prior history revealed an episode of cholecystitis four years ago. She had avoided taking anything for the headaches until she took two Tylenol just before calling for the ambulance.

Physical exam revealed little new information. Together with the swelling in her hands and feet, Janice's face seemed quite puffy. Although the fetal heart rate was difficult to monitor, she indicated that the babies were quite active.

Vital signs revealed an apprehensive, yet alert mother, with pupils equal and reactive, pulse 88 regular and strong, respiration 24 and regular, blood pressure 180/108, skin pale with peripheral edema. The ECG showed a normal sinus rhythm.

During questioning, Janice stated she had her blood pressure taken at her last doctor's appointment, and there was no mention of anything out of the norm. After being reassured she was in good hands, she was assisted to the stretcher, placed in the left lateral recumbent position, and provided with a high concentration of oxygen. An IV, with normal saline, was started at a TKO rate.

En route, a second set of vitals was obtained and a call to the receiving hospital was initiated relaying the following information: alert thirty-six-year-old female in her thirty-fourth week of gestation with twins, complaining of headache, blurred vision, and abdominal pain; vital signs include pulse 90 regular, respirations 24 and blood pressure 188/114.

En route, Janice complained of an increased intensity with regard to her headache and, as a result, the paramedics kept the lights low and managed to avoid using the siren. They were concerned that the complication they were dealing with might be toxemia of pregnancy (preeclampsia) and therefore hoped to reduce external stimuli, which might precipitate a seizure.

Multiple-Choice Questions

1. Regarding the fetus, which of the following statements are true?
   1. Fetal movements start approximately the thirtieth week of gestation.
   2. Fetal movements start approximately the twentieth week of gestation.
   3. Fetal heart sounds become audible approximately the thirtieth week of gestation.
   4. Fetal heart sounds become audible approximately the twentieth week of gestation.
      a) 1, 3
      b) 1, 4
      c) 2, 3
      d) 2, 4
      e) none of the above

2. The normal weight gain during pregnancy along with the increase in circulating blood volume means that:

1. An increase in pulse rate of 10 to 20 beats is not unusual.
2. An increase in pulse rate of 20 to 30 beats is not unusual.
3. Hypertension during pregnancy is rarely a concern.
4. Hypotension during pregnancy is rarely a concern.

   a) 1
   b) 1, 3
   c) 2, 4
   d) 1, 3, 4
   e) 2, 3, 4

3. When distinguishing between true and false labor, it is important to remember:

1. True labor pains may often be relieved by walking.
2. Increases in the intensity of true labor pain are usually incremental.
3. During false labor the frequency of contractions is commonly irregular.
4. During false labor the duration or length of contractions is usually consistent.

   a) 1, 3
   b) 2, 4
   c) 2, 3
   d) 1, 3, 4
   e) 2, 3, 4

4. Toxemia of pregnancy, a condition still considered idiopathic, is:

1. seen more frequently in women over thirty
2. a risk factor for women with pre-existing heart disease
3. a risk factor among diabetic women
4. seen more frequently in women under twenty

   a) 1, 2, 3
   b) 1, 2, 4
   c) 1, 3, 4
   d) 2, 3, 4
   e) all of the above

5. Suspected factors contributing to the development of toxemia of pregnancy include:

1. poor economic status
2. poor nutritional intake

3. inadequate prenatal care
4. recent immigration

   a) 1, 2
   b) 2, 3
   c) 1, 2, 3
   d) 2, 3, 4
   e) 1, 3, 4

6. Toxemia of pregnancy results in a generalized vasospasm of unknown origin and is divided into two categories:

1. preeclampsia defined as hypotension associated with generalized dehydration
2. preeclampsia defined as hypertension associated with peripheral edema
3. eclampsia defined as a partial seizure associated with pregnancy-induced hypotension
4. eclampsia defined as tonic-clonic seizures associated with pregnancy-induced hypertension

   a) 1, 4
   b) 1, 3
   c) 2, 4
   d) 2, 3
   e) none of the above

7. Eclampsia can be a life-threatening disease to both the mother and her unborn child, therefore, early detection is very important. Weight gain needs to be closely monitored and should not average more than _____ per week during the third trimester:

a) .5 lbs
b) 1 lb
c) 1.5 lbs
d) 2 lbs
e) 2.5 lbs

8. The onset of toxemia of pregnancy:

1. occurs most often in the second trimester
2. occurs most often in the third trimester
3. is often insidious and may be asymptomatic
4. usually results in edema first, followed by hypertension

   a) 1, 3
   b) 2, 4
   c) 2, 3
   d) 1, 3, 4
   e) 2, 3, 4

9. Signs and symptoms most often associated with toxemia of pregnancy include:

1. visual disturbances
2. tinnitus
3. hypotension
4. facial edema

    a) 1, 3
    b) 1, 4
    c) 2, 3
    d) 2, 3, 4
    e) 1, 2, 4

10. Signs and symptoms commonly associated with toxemia of pregnancy include:

1. epigastric abdominal pain
2. oliguria
3. swollen hands
4. hypertension

    a) 1, 4
    b) 1, 2
    c) 1, 3, 4
    d) 2, 3, 4
    e) all of the above

11. Complications that could result from eclampsia include:

1. intracranial hemorrhage
2. abruptio placentae
3. seizures
4. pulmonary edema

    a) 1, 2, 3
    b) 1, 2, 4
    c) 1, 3, 4
    d) 2, 3, 4
    e) all of the above

12. Management of the patient with severe preeclampsia may include:

1. reducing external stimuli to minimize CNS excitability
2. hyperventilation of the patient in order to decrease cerebral edema
3. provision of a high oxygen concentration to minimize the risk of hypoxia
4. preparing for potential seizure activity

    a) 2, 3
    b) 1, 4

c)   1, 2, 3
d)   1, 3, 4
e)   2, 3, 4

Debriefing

Often the paramedic in the field finds only one or two well-defined signs or symptoms. There is no opportunity to draw blood and send it to the lab for analysis, no x-rays or scans, and no specialists to call on. Yet, despite this lack of assistance, or perhaps because of it, the paramedic must pay close attention to any signs and symptoms that suggest serious complications in an otherwise non-threatening situation.

A keen sense of observation and good listening skills may be all that is required to give a proper priority to the call. The call in this particular case deserved the highest priority for there could be life-threatening consequences for both mother and babies.

As obstetric calls go, this case did not meet the criteria for imminent delivery, since there were no regularly defined contractions, her water (amniotic fluid) had not broken, there was no stated desire to push or bear down, and she was still six weeks away from term. In addition, there were no signs of bleeding, which might point to other serious third-trimester complications such as placenta previa or abruptio placentae. Vital signs did not indicate that she was in shock. Why then the cause for concern?

Preeclampsia syndrome is a group of symptoms associated with late pregnancy. As a syndrome the exact nature or etiology of the disease is idiopathic. Preeclampsia, also known as toxemia of pregnancy (it was once believed that a toxin was produced by the mother in reaction to a foreign protein of the fetus), is characterized by edema, proteinuria, and hypertension. Eclampsia itself describes the severe late stage of this disease and is characterized by seizure activity.

Pathological changes in the glomeruli of the kidney produce proteinuria and diminished urine output. The reduction in glomerular filtration, combined with an increased sodium reabsorption, causes fluid retention and edema. Normal weight gain approximates one pound a week in the third trimester; any more should be noted. Some ankle edema is also normal, but in the case of toxemia of pregnancy there is often a marked swelling of the upper body, particularly a puffiness of the face and hands.

The second major sign is hypertension, and is usually acknowledged if the patient's blood pressure is greater than 140/90. As the blood pressure creeps higher there is an ensuing risk of convulsions on the part of the expectant mother.

Other symptoms that signal a move toward the eclamptic stage include fever, headache, blurred vision, and epigastric pain. These are warning signs of increasing cerebral edema and CNS irritability and should not be ignored by paramedics. Once these signs are recognized, they should transport the patient to the hospital immediately.

The danger that seizures present includes a significant risk of cerebral hypoxia for both mother and babies (in this case twins). Complications for the babies result mostly from prematurity, since, in the eclamptic stage, once convulsions are under control, the babies are almost always delivered.

In this particular presentation, Janice had a prior history of cholecystitis, so the diagnosis would seem appropriate, if not for the peripheral edema and high blood pressure. It is always best to err on the side of caution, bringing the patient in without delay even if the diagnosis turns out to be an inflamed gallbladder. The fact that there was no prior history of hypertension during her visits to the doctor does not negate the possibility of toxemia, since it is often insidious, arising acutely and without prior warning.

Notifying the receiving hospital should be a requirement on all priority calls so that the staff can be prepared. The importance is obvious in this situation.

Follow-Up

Mrs. Forest arrived at the emergency room and was seen immediately. Once assessed she was diagnosed with severe preeclampsia and given an intravenous infusion of magnesium sulfate to promote fluid excretion, reduce blood pressure, and forestall convulsive seizures. Since this drug is a CNS depressant, she received constant monitoring, assessing deep tendon reflexes and respirations. Urinary output was also monitored every four hours to ensure that a minimum of 100 ml was being excreted over the four-hour period to avoid magnesium toxicity, since this mineral is excreted almost exclusively in the urine.

Mrs. Forest delivered the same day by caesarean section two fraternal boys weighing 4.8 pounds (2200 grams) each. The premature nature of the births manifested itself in hyaline membrane disease and liver immaturity for which they were treated and closely monitored in the neonatal intensive care unit.

Fact from Fiction

Pregnancy-induced hyertension (PIH), which includes toxemia of pregnancy, more appropriately called preeclampsia/eclampsia, has as yet an uncertain etiology. The preeclampsia form of PIH is characterized by salt and water retention by the kidneys, weight gain, and edema especially of the face and hands.

The best accepted theory relates to abnormal synthesis of prostaglandins and thromboxanes which act as vasoconstrictors on the systemic circulation. Adverse systemic vasoconstriction leads to decreased perfusion of maternal organ systems, and includes the fetus and placenta. Arterial spasm occurs in many organs, including the kidneys, liver, and, most important, the brain. Seizure activity is caused by cerebral vasospasm. Renal hypoxia results in increased glomerular permeability and a loss of protein from the vascular system. The resultant decrease in colloid osmotic pressure allows for a fluid shift from intravascular to interstitial, which accounts for edema and weight gain. Oliguria and proteinuria are two clinical effects of renal compromise.

As arterial tension increases severely (extreme hypertension), clinical features include headache, visual disturbances, and confusion. Magnesium sulfate is used to prevent and treat seizures since it blocks calcium uptake by neurons without producing generalized nervous system depression in the mother and fetus.

Prognosis and outcome depend on the severity of signs and symptoms. Hypertension crisis concluding with tonic-clonic convulsions can result in cerebral hemorrhage in mom and physiologic shock to the fetus. Induction of labor and delivery of the infant is necessitated when the life of the mother and/or the fetus is in imminent danger. Caesarean section has reduced mortality rates significantly, however, early recognition, as in most diseases leading to emergencies, is still the key to a favorable outcome.

Answer Key & Rationale

1. d) Babies born before the twentieth week of gestation are generally not considered viable. Few of those born between the twentieth and thirtieth week will survive. The longer the gestation, the better the chances. Fetal heart rate and movements may be heard and felt after the twentieth week of gestation.

2. a) The normal weight gain for the expectant mother is approximately twenty-four pounds to term. An associated increase in heart rate of fifteen heartbeats per minute is the norm toward the end of the third trimester. There is also an increase of approximately thirty percent in overall blood volume.

Hypertension is always a concern since it may signal toxemia of pregnancy. Hypotension is also a concern as it may be indicative of internal hemorrhage.

3. c) In true labor the contractions are regular in both frequency and duration. The intensity of contractions steadily increases toward delivery.

In false labor the contractions may be very irregular. For example, they may come at intervals of five, eight, and two minutes, and last for varying lengths of time, such as twenty, ten, or thirty seconds.

4. e) Toxemia of pregnancy is seen most frequently in younger women and older women experiencing their first pregnancies. Risk factors (although no causal relationship has been established) include obesity, diabetes, heart disease, renal disease, and chronic hypertension. There is also a greater occurrence among those with multiple births or polyhydramnios.

5. b) Factors suspected to contribute to a predisposition to toxemia of pregnancy include a lack of prenatal care and inadequate dietary intake, especially in regard to protein. Social and economic factors are not directly related to the predisposition to preeclampsia. Indirectly, however, a lack of income might lead to poor nutrition.

6. c) Toxemia of pregnancy is divided into two general stages, preeclampsia and eclampsia. They are both associated with hypertension, the preeclamptic being the early stage characterized by peripheral edema and proteinuria, while the eclamptic stage represents a critically ill patient with tonic-clonic convulsions, which can potentially lead to coma and death.

7. b) Sudden weight gain should always signal concern; however, where normal weight gain can be one to two pounds a week in the second trimester, the third trimester should see weight gain of no more than a pound a week.

8. e) Toxemia of pregnancy occurs most often in the third trimester and frequently without warning. The patient may be unaware of the seriousness of the disease since the early signs of rapid weight gain and peripheral edema are not usually alarming. Medical attention may not be sought until other signs of severe preeclampsia establish themselves.

9. b); 10. e) Signs and symptoms associated with toxemia of pregnancy include visual disturbances, headache, epigastric pain, disorientation, oliguria, hypertension, swollen hands, facial puffiness, and diffuse peripheral edema. Seizures leading to coma are the late stages of the disease process.

11. e) Eclampsia is the life-threatening stage and may result in intracranial hemorrhage, internal hemorrhage from abruptio placentae secondary to seizures, and pulmonary edema from increased hydrostatic pressure secondary to hypertension and renal failure.

12. d) Definitive treatment in this case is management of seizures and delivery of the fetus. Rapid transport is therefore indicated, keeping lights low and reducing the noise level to minimize external stress on the central nervous system. Provision of a high concentration of oxygen, and placement of the patient in the left lateral decubitus position to decrease the risk of uterine pressure on the vena cava, and to promote airway management in case of vomiting. Preparing for seizures means employing safety measures to minimize the risk of injury to the patient, as well as having suction equipment available and ready for use.

Hyperventilation will not be very effective in reducing cerebral edema since the edema has not resulted from a buildup of carbon dioxide leading to cerebral vasodilation. Cerebral edema may be partially compensated for by elevating the head 15 to 30 degrees in order to promote cerebral venous drainage. Hyperventilation may be helpful in the eclamptic stage if the patient has sustained cerebral hypoxia resulting from prolonged seizure activity.

CASE STUDY 8

A light snow had just begun to sift downward when a 911 call came in for an eighteen-year-old female with difficulty breathing. The paramedics proceeded on the highest priority level, knowing it could be anything from anxiety-induced hyperventilation to a life-threatening dyspnea secondary to a disease process such as cystic fibrosis, multiple sclerosis, or a myasthenia gravis crisis.

The apartment building had only four floors and looked as if in need of repair. Tracy Fraser opened the door to her second-floor apartment and immediately returned inside to sit down. She sat on the edge of the sofa and leaned forward, drawing each breath with obvious effort. Tracy said that she shared the apartment with a girlfriend and would have had her roommate drive her to hospital but she was working.

It was mid-afternoon and Tracy said she had been out grocery shopping and had just arrived back when her breathing problems began. Tracy stated that she had been asthmatic since childhood and that she had taken four puffs of her Ventolin five minutes apart today, but was still experiencing shortness of breath. One of the paramedics checked that the date on the inhaler had not expired and noticed that the recommended dosage was one to two puffs.

They quickly set up the oxygen equipment and provided Tracy with 100 percent oxygen via nonrebreather mask at 12 lpm. An IV with normal saline was also inserted. Her breathing pattern represented a combination of tachypnea with hypopnea. In the management of her dyspnea, they encouraged her to slow her rate of breathing by exhaling for a prolonged period and to increase her volume by breathing in deeply.

During the investigation into the cause, she stated that she hadn't had an attack since early fall, which was over four months ago, and had managed the episode successfully with her inhaler. She was a first-year student in business administration and had been stressed out with midterms for much of the week but was feeling better, having just finished her last test yesterday.

She denied any medical history other than asthma, did not abuse drugs, had no food allergies that she was aware of, and had not eaten since early that morning. She admitted to being a smoker and was smoking at the time her dyspnea started. There were painters in the stairwells whose work had just commenced that day, and Tracy believed that the fumes from the paint, which permeated the building, may have triggered her asthma attack.

A quick physical assessment revealed retractions and the use of accessory muscles in order to breathe. No visible rashes were present to suggest anaphylaxis. There were audible wheezes during expiration and air entry could be auscultated throughout the chest with diminished sounds bilaterally in the lower lobes. Rales/crackles were absent and there was no indication of a recent illness or trauma.

Vital signs revealed a pulse, which was 94 regular and strong, respirations 28 shallow and labored, blood pressure 118/76, pupils equal and reactive, skin cool and color pale. Pulse oximetry revealed an oxygen saturation of 75 percent. The ECG showed a normal sinus rhythm. Tracy continued to receive coaching on her breathing pattern, particularly to maintain an extended expiratory phase.

Tracy met the protocol for albuterol administration and verbal consent was obtained. A 2.5 mg nebule was added to the nebulizer mask and the flow rate adjusted to 8 lpm.

Tracy had waited a good half hour before calling for help, which meant that this episode had now lasted close to an hour, with little hope that it would resolve itself on its own. She was also upset at the superintendent for not putting up notices of painting to be done in the building. Tracy was speaking in short, choppy sentences with increasing effort and was starting to take on an exhausted appearance.

The paramedics had worked quickly. Total time at scene was less than ten minutes before Tracy was prepared for transport. She was placed in a Fowler position and the high concentration of humidified oxygen, initiated on arrival, was continued.

En route, her coughing, which had been sporadic at the scene, was now becoming quite frequent and productive. Tracy, who had been very communicative at the scene, was now no longer talking but was concentrating totally on breathing.

A second auscultation of the lung fields revealed a much quieter chest bilaterally and peripheral cyanosis could be observed on her lips. Rapid consult with the receiving hospital alerted the emergency staff to the patient's condition: severe respiratory distress resulting from an asthma attack.

A second dose of 2.5 mg of albuterol was given by nebulizer, since Tracy's dyspnea was increasing and an obvious ventilation-perfusion imbalance was developing.

Multiple-Choice Questions

1. Which of the following statements relating to asthma are true?
   1. It is a condition involving episodic periods of bronchospasm.
   2. Most attacks are chronic with very little freedom from symptoms between episodes.
   3. It is not possible, as it was once believed, to outgrow childhood asthma.
   4. It occurs in families, suggesting a predisposition to genetic transmission.

   a) 1, 2
   b) 1, 4
   c) 2, 3
   d) 1, 3, 4
   e) 2, 3, 4

2. When comparing extrinsic to intrinsic asthma, which of the following characteristics can be differentiated?
   1. The age of onset for extrinsic asthma is usually under thirty-five.
   2. Allergies are generally absent in intrinsic asthma.
   3. Intrinsic asthma is often seasonal.
   4. A family history of allergies is more common in extrinsic asthma.

   a) 1, 3
   b) 1, 4
   c) 2, 3
   d) 1, 2, 4
   e) 2, 3, 4

3. Factors common to most types of asthma include:
   1. interaction of antibodies with red blood cell-bound IgE molecules
   2. bronchial smooth muscle spasm
   3. inflammation of mucous membranes
   4. increased production of surfactant around alveoli

   a) 1, 4
   b) 1, 2
   c) 2, 3
   d) 1, 3, 4
   e) 2, 3, 4

4. The ventilation-perfusion mismatch created during an asthma attack can result in:
   1. hypoxemia
   2. early respiratory alkalosis

3. metabolic alkalosis
4. late respiratory acidosis

    a) 2, 4
    b) 1, 2
    c) 2, 3
    d) 1, 3, 4
    e) 1, 2, 4

5. Clinical manifestations relating to acute asthma include:

1. symptoms that are present even during periods of remission
2. dyspnea and increased work of breathing
3. audible rales/crackles throughout the lungs
4. wheezing particularly evident on expiration

    a) 2, 4
    b) 1, 3
    c) 1, 2
    d) 2, 3, 4
    e) 1, 3, 4

6. Severe attacks of asthma are often accompanied by:

1. use of the accessory muscles of respiration
2. a productive cough
3. tachycardia and tachypnea
4. stridor and hoarseness

    a) 1, 4
    b) 2, 4
    c) 1, 2, 4
    d) 1, 2, 3
    e) 2, 3, 4

7. Status asthmaticus is a life-threatening situation, which does not respond to normal treatment and can often be associated with:

1. pneumothorax
2. paradoxical pulse
3. hemothorax
4. absent air sounds

    a) 1, 4
    b) 2, 3
    c) 3, 4
    d) 1, 2, 4
    e) 1, 2, 3

8. Complications that can result from repeated bouts of asthma may include:
1. pulmonary emboli
2. pulmonary edema
3. atelectasis
4. pneumonia
   a) 1, 2
   b) 1, 3
   c) 3, 4
   d) 1, 2, 4
   e) 2, 3, 4

9. Asthmatic attacks may be provoked by a variety of stimuli such as:
1. vigorous exertion
2. smoke
3. atmospheric pollutants
4. pollens
   a) 1, 2, 3
   b) 1, 2, 4
   c) 1, 3, 4
   d) 2, 3, 4
   e) all of the above

10. Cyanosis, diaphoresis, agitation, somnolence, and confusion may all be associated with a severe episode of asthma and result from:
1. hypoxia
2. hypertension
3. hypercapnia
4. exhaustion
   a) 1, 3
   b) 2, 3
   c) 2, 4
   d) 1, 3, 4
   e) 1, 2, 4

11. Bronchodilators commonly used in the treatment of asthmatics include:
1. epinephrine
2. corticosteroids
3. albuterol
4. aminophylline
   a) 2, 4
   b) 1, 3, 4
   c) 1, 2, 3
   d) 2, 3, 4
   e) all of the above

12. Which of the following general statements relating to asthma are correct?
1. Due to ever-increasing advances in medicine, the number of asthma sufferers is on the decline.
2. Most people who develop asthma do so during childhood.
3. Treatment of an attack is geared toward eliminating the causative agents while reversing bronchospasm and airway obstruction.
4. Skin tests will positively identify the causal agent and, once it is found, immunization in the form of vaccines can be given.

   a) 2, 3
   b) 2, 4
   c) 1, 3
   d) 1, 2, 4
   e) 1, 3, 4

Debriefing

Some calls can be sized up simply with good observation skills and a little experience. In this case, as in many with respiratory compromise, the patient was sitting forward on the edge of the couch, probably with hands on knees, while making an exaggerated effort to both talk and breathe. This position (leaning forward with arms extended outward) reflects true orthopnea and is a classic sign of respiratory distress. It can be seen in a child with acute epiglottitis, as well as an elderly person with emphysema. Other important clues include the use of accessory muscles, which come into play when the diaphragm starts to tire. Retractions around the neck and clavicles is the sign to look for.

When determining the cause of respiratory distress, it is important to stop and consider that most people suffering an attack of asthma have had numerous previous episodes and a long association with the disease. Most patients are aware of what will likely trigger an attack (in this case, paint fumes), so listen attentively to their story. Environmental allergies and the number of asthma sufferers are on the rise.

If metered-dose inhalers such as albuterol, a beta-agonist, are used but do not provide relief, then it is likely additional treatment will be required to arrest the attack. It is often helpful for the paramedics to carry a pocket-sized drug book with them. In this case they already knew that the drug albuterol (Ventolin), relieves bronchospasm, is most often used to prevent exercise-induced asthma, and has the potential to cause certain side effects including nausea, headache, tachycardia, hypertension, tremors, and dizziness.

Treatment should not be delayed in any case of respiratory compromise, so the crew in this case quickly provided oxygen. It is important not to wait until a complete assessment has been made since hypoxemia will probably be well established by the time help arrives, and hypoxia will be following closely behind. A high concentration of humidified oxygen is the preferred treatment, even with patients suffering from chronic obstructive pulmonary disease (COPD). The hypoxic drive of patients with COPD simply means that EMTs must watch the respiratory rate vigilantly. If the rate falls too low, then supplemental manual ventilations will have to be provided.

Unfortunately, most portable oxygen devices are not humidified; humidity can help loosen up the phlegm clogging the bronchioles. In addition, many asthma patients may sense a further constriction if forced to use a face mask. A nasal canula provides only about half the concentration, but it is better than going without. One of the best management intervention techniques in the treatment of acute asthma is to coach the patient to extend the expiratory phase of the respiratory cycle. First the stale air, trapped in alveoli behind clogged and spasmed bronchioles, must be allowed to escape. Only then can fresh air enter.

Management of the asthmatic is based on gaining a better ventilation-perfusion balance. The anxiety of fighting for breath induces tachypnea, but a slower respiratory rate with a prolonged expiration and deeper inhalation helps far more in gaining a better air exchange. A high Fowler position aids the descent of the diaphragm and allows for maximum lung expansion.

Albuterol (Ventolin, Salbutamol) the medication of choice for acute asthma, is classified as a bronchodilator and sympathomimetic. It relaxes the smooth muscles of the bronchial tree by stimulating beta-adrenergic receptors of the sympathetic nervous system. Most asthma sufferers will experience relief through the nebulizer within three to ten minutes. In severe cases of asthma one dose may not be enough.

Coughing is a common symptom associated with acute asthma and is often dry in the early stages, but as time progresses, mucus will be brought up. As mentioned earlier, humidified oxygen will help break up the mucus and ease breathing. It is important to note that the work required to breathe during an asthma attack often quadruples, with the patient gradually becoming dehydrated and exhausted. Therefore, the patient should rest as much as possible.

The lungs may not be uniformly obstructed and auscultation of all major lobes is important since a "quiet chest" does not mean that the symptoms have abated. Just the opposite is true: it could indicate an absence of air movement that could become life threatening. As seen in this case, Tracy's condition deteriorated en route. Monitoring of her air entry, level of consciousness, and presence of cyanosis were all crucial since preparations had to be made for a respiratory arrest situation.

Follow-Up

On arrival at the emergency room, Tracy was taken into the "resuscitation room" and treated aggressively in order to regain an adequate perfusion/ventilation ratio. An acute asthma attack was confirmed as the diagnosis. The IV started in the field was used for rehydration, and she received Ventolin and Atrovent inhalation therapy, as well as epinephrine after being placed on a cardiac monitor.

Tracy recovered over the course of the evening and did not have to stay overnight. She was encouraged to increase her fluid intake and she stayed at her parents' place during the following week until the painting in her apartment building was completed.

Fact from Fiction

Asthma is defined as recurring episode of wheezing and dyspnea resulting from spasmodic contractions of the bronchi and bronchioles. A key point to remember is its reversibility.

There are a number of etiologies that categorize asthma, including: extrinsic asthma; intrinsic asthma; exercise-induced asthma; occupationally induced asthma; drug-induced asthma; and cardiac asthma.

Extrinsic asthma accounts for up to half of all cases and is common in children and young adults. There is often a positive family history and it is associated with hay fever, dust allergies, animal dander, and positive skin test reactions to allergens.

The antigen–IgE antibody response results in the release of inflammatory chemicals from mast cells in the airways. Degranulation of mast cells and release of bradykinine, cytokines, and other bronchoactive mediators produce the clinical features of an acute attack.

Intrinsic asthma frequently develops in adulthood after age thirty-five and with the causative factors being less well defined. It often appears in conjunction with respiratory infections and attacks of this type can be quite severe.

Exercise-induced asthma often occurs five to ten minutes after the exercise has begun. Bronchospasms from smooth muscle contractions occur as an increased rate and depth of breathing lead to a cooling and dehydration of the lower airways. Symptoms seem to occur more rapidly in cold weather. Providing humidified oxygen in most asthmatic episodes gives some relief.

Occupational asthma is associated with exposure to allergens and various toxins whose fumes come from any number of sources in the work environment. Since most do not produce skin reactions, testing to prove hypersensitivity is difficult.

Drug-induced asthma is most often associated with aspirin and other non-steroidal anti-inflammatories such as ibuprofen or indomethacin. Sensitized patients with asthma, nasal polyps, or sinusitis are particularly at risk for a severe or potentially fatal asthma attack if they ingest aspirin. Associated symptoms can include a decrease in blood pressure, itching, rhinorrhea, or a rash.

Cardiac asthma is the result of bronchospasm precipitated by congestive heart failure.

Despite the categorization above, it is important to note that asthma is a multifactorial disease and not only may have more than one cause, but follows more than one pathogenic mechanism.

Answer Key & Rationale

1. b) Asthma gives rise to periods of spasm or prolonged contraction of the lung's bronchial smooth muscle. Most attacks are short-lived, with freedom from symptoms and complete recovery between episodes. There is a hereditary tendency to develop asthma, although the mode of genetic transmission is unclear.

About half of all sufferers of childhood asthma will have resolved their disease by the time of puberty.

2. d) Asthma is characterized as extrinsic if it is triggered by allergens and intrinsic if it is not. Extrinsic asthma results in those who are highly sensitized to antigens such as dust and pollens, or it develops from prolonged exposure to irritants. This type of asthma develops in those under the age of thirty-five, is often seasonal in nature, and is associated with a family history of allergies.

Intrinsic asthma has no known immunologic cause, and usually occurs in adults over thirty-five years of age who are sensitive to aspirin and have nasal polyps. This type of asthma also seems to occur in patients with a history of recurrent bronchial or sinus infections.

3. c) Hypersensitivity of the airways is common to all types of asthma and is related to the interaction of an antigen (not antibody) with mast cell-bound IgE molecules that produce an immediate inflammatory response of bronchial smooth muscle spasm, edema, bronchial constriction, and a thick tenacious mucus. (A mast cell is a type of white blood cell.) There is also a resultant increase in the number and size of mucus-producing glands.

4. e) The result of poor air exchange during acute asthma leads to hypoxemia as some areas of the lungs are not adequately providing the pulmonary vasculature with oxygen. Respiratory alkalosis results as hyperventilation is triggered to compensate for decreased ventilation. As the obstruction worsens over time, carbon dioxide is retained, creating respiratory acidosis. Hypoxemia then creates hypoxia and metabolic acidosis.

5. a) Signs and symptoms of acute asthma include a tightness in the chest with an increased internal lung pressure. The actual work to exchange gasses during an attack can increase tenfold. Wheezes, which are high-pitched musical sounds, can be heard over both lung fields during both phases of respiration, or on exhalation only. Audible wheezes result when air is forced through the narrowed and constricted bronchioles.

Rales/crackles and associated pulmonary edema are not common signs of acute asthma.

Although pulmonary function tests may reveal some abnormality, patients with asthma can be completely asymptomatic between attacks.

6. d) The patient with an acute episode of asthma most often presents sitting and leaning forward with hands on the knees. As the diaphragm (the major respiratory muscle) tires, accessory muscles are brought into play in order to carry on the work of breathing.

A dry cough is seen in the early stages while a productive cough with a thick tenacious mucus is seen in more prolonged bouts.

The combination of anxiety and hypoxemia result in an increased respiratory and heart rate.

Stridor and hoarseness are seen most often with an upper respiratory obstruction, whereas asthma is considered a lower airway obstruction.

7. d) Status asthmaticus can be life threatening, since any prolonged asthma attack will eventually lead to exhaustion, hypoxia, and respiratory failure. Air flow may be so reduced that wheezing can no longer be heard. The absent air sounds or "quiet chest" signals eminent danger. As air pressure increases behind the obstructed bronchioles, a pneumothorax or atelectasis may develop. As well, intrathoracic pressure may rise to the point where the pulse is felt to be weaker on inspiration and stronger during expiration (pulsus paradoxus).

Since trauma is not usually part of the history, hemothorax associated with asthma is very rare.

8. c) Completely obstructed bronchioles may result in atelectasis and pneumonia. Pulmonary edema may follow the pneumonia, and as such is only indirectly related to asthma. Pulmonary emboli are not commonly associated with asthma attacks.

9. e) Acute asthma may be exercise-induced. These attacks are usually preventable with the use of a bronchodilator before exercising. Noxious fumes such as smoke, paint, or other gasses may trigger an attack. Environmental changes in humidity and temperature may give rise to an onset of acute asthma. Emotional stress can be the event that brings on an episode of acute asthma. The instigating event or allergen may also be of unknown origin.

10. d) As the patient tires from the effort needed to exchange gases, hypoxia and hypercapnia build toward a state of metabolic acidosis, which in turn depresses the CNS. Signs and symptoms of shock may all be evidenced in the late stages of an unresolved asthma attack.

11. b) Epinephrine (Bronkaid Mist; Primatene Mist), albuterol (Proventil; Ventolin), and aminophylline (Corophyllin, Lixaminol) are used to dilate bronchioles. Corticosteroids may be used in the treatment and prevention of asthma; however, their benefit comes mainly from their anti-inflammatory effects.

12. a) The type of asthma seen early in life is the extrinsic variety. Childhood asthma accounts for 50 percent of all cases while another 30 percent of sufferers are under the age of thirty-five.

Treatment of asthma is aimed at eliminating the cause or removing the patient from the environment that contains the allergen, and reversing bronchospasm and bronchiole obstruction in order to create a proper ventilation and perfusion ratio.

There is no immunization for asthma and, despite advances in medicine, the number of asthma sufferers is on the rise.

CASE STUDY 9

911 RESPONSE: sixty-six-year-old female with shortness of breath

It was early Sunday morning in the city: 1:30 A.M., and the streets had finally been emptied of Saturday night revelers. Just as the calm was descending, a 911 call registered a woman sixty-six years old with difficulty breathing. The crew arrived in minutes because the traffic was sparse and the address given led them to a nearby seniors' building.

The paramedics piled the jump kit, portable oxygen, portable suction, and a defibrillator/cardiac monitor onto the stretcher. Once inside the building they found themselves confronted with an "out of order" service elevator and a passenger elevator too small to accommodate their stretcher. Even with the gurney seated upright and length compressed to the smallest size the elevator was not big enough.

The attending paramedic went up alone while the second crew member stayed to prepare the stretcher outside the elevator before going up with a stair chair.

On arrival at the inevitable "last apartment down the hallway on the right," the paramedic found Mrs. Atwater living alone and visibly distressed. She was ambulatory and, after letting the paramedic in, slowly made her way back to a kitchen chair. Between breaths in which audible congestion could be heard, Mrs. Atwater stated she'd recently been widowed, her husband having died of prostate cancer three months earlier. When asked what initiated her call, Mrs. Atwater related she hadn't felt well all evening, and thought perhaps she was coming down with a cold. Her family, which included a number of grandchildren, had been over for Thanksgiving dinner. She felt she might have overdone it, and become too tired.

The paramedic listened empathetically while setting up the oxygen equipment and then, while providing a high concentration through a non-rebreather mask, tried to get Mrs. Atwater to focus on what appeared to be her chief complaint by asking what had brought on the respiratory distress.

She didn't know why she was having a breathing problem. She had simply gone to bed around eleven-thirty after cleaning up and was awakened at one o'clock unable to breathe. Previous history revealed adult onset diabetes for which she was taking hypoglycemics. She was obese; however, there was no history of high blood pressure, and no complaints of any heart ailment of any kind in the past. She did not smoke and consumed alcohol in very moderate amounts.

Physical examination revealed a significant amount of rales/crackles auscultated bilaterally throughout the lung bases. Skin condition was pale, cool, and diaphoretic. There was no evidence of pitting edema to extremities, no ascites recorded, and jugular vein distention was not noticeable. Auscultation of heart sounds was unremarkable.

On reassessment, Mrs. Atwater stated that although she still felt very weak, she was able to breath much easier since being up and that the oxygen was also helping. Vital signs revealed an alert, coherent elderly women with pulse 110 regular but weak; respirations 26 and labored; blood pressure 138/104; and pupils equal and reactive. Mrs. Atwater was without cough or fever and had otherwise no recent medical complaints until this morning.

She seemed somewhat depressed and described her present condition by saying that it had all been "a bit too much last night" and that perhaps she had "just run out of gas."

By now the second crew member had arrived. The cardiac monitor was attached and was showing sinus tachycardia. A IV was inserted with normal saline TKO. The paramedics explained the stair chair to Mrs. Atwater, wrapped her warmly, reassured her, and transported her to the stretcher waiting in the lobby. A second set of vitals showed orthostatic changes in heart rate, blood pressure, and decreasing LOC characterized by confusion with increased anxiety.

Once in the ambulance, the paramedics began the process of dealing with the pulmonary edema. Initially, they administered 0.4 mg SL of NTG. They followed the NTG with Lasix 40 mg IV. Mrs. Atwater was then transported in the Fowler position and the hospital was notified en route. The chief complaint was given as pulmonary edema possibly secondary to heart failure.

Multiple-Choice Questions

1. Left-sided heart failure is commonly called:
1. congestive heart failure
2. cor pulmonale
3. left ventricular failure
4. pulmonary edema
   a) 1, 2
   b) 1, 3
   c) 2, 4
   d) 1, 3, 4
   e) 2, 3, 4

2. The two most common causes of left heart failure extrinsic to the myocardium are:

   1. myocardial infarction
   2. systemic hypertension
   3. aortic stenosis and regurgitation
   4. pernicious anemia

      a) 1, 4
      b) 2, 4
      c) 2, 3
      d) 1, 3
      e) 1, 2

3. The presence of pulmonary edema in heart failure indicates:

   1. decreased pressure in the pulmonary capillaries
   2. decreased pressure in the right ventricle
   3. increased pressure in the left atrium
   4. increased pressure in the pulmonary vein

      a) 1, 2
      b) 2, 4
      c) 1, 3
      d) 3, 4
      e) 2, 3

4. The onset of heart failure in women often presents with two classic findings:

   1. orthopnea
   2. stabbing chest pain
   3. heart palpitations
   4. paroxysmal nocturnal dyspnea

      a) 1, 2
      b) 1, 3
      c) 2, 3
      d) 2, 4
      e) 1, 4

5. Acute pulmonary edema develops when:

   1. right-sided heart failure occurs
   2. pulmonary capillary hydrostatic pressure is high
   3. increased capillary permeability exists
   4. left-sided heart failure occurs

      a) 1, 4
      b) 1, 2
      c) 3, 4
      d) 2, 3, 4
      e) 1, 2, 3

6. Signs and symptoms associated with pulmonary edema include:
   1. hypoxemia
   2. tachypnea
   3. crackles and wheezes
   4. dysphagia
      a) 1, 2, 3
      b) 1, 2, 4
      c) 1, 3, 4
      d) 2, 3, 4
      e) all of the above

7. Signs and symptoms associated with pulmonary edema include:
   1. dyspnea
   2. frothy sputum
   3. fever
   4. anxiety
      a) 1, 2, 3
      b) 1, 3, 4
      c) 1, 2, 4
      d) 2, 3, 4
      e) all of the above

8. Non-cardiogenic causes of pulmonary edema include:
   1. inhalation injury
   2. aspiration pneumonia
   3. near drowning
   4. narcotic overdose
   5. septic shock
   6. high-altitude exertion
      a) 1, 2, 4, 6
      b) 2, 3, 5, 6
      c) 1, 2, 3, 4, 5
      d) 1, 3, 4, 5, 6
      e) all of the above

9. Management of a patient in acute pulmonary edema includes:
   1. improving gas exchange with high oxygen concentration
   2. increased venous return with elevation of extremities
   3. reducing anxiety by reassurance and explanation of procedures
   4. maximizing ventilation with Fowler positioning
      a) 1, 2, 3
      b) 1, 2, 4

c) 2, 3, 4
d) 1, 3, 4
e) all of the above

10. Sympathetic nervous system response to congestive heart failure leads to increased:

1. heart rate and myocardial oxygen demand
2. cardiac output and blood pressure
3. urinary output relieving fluid overload
4. peripheral vasoconstriction promoting venous return

    a) 1, 3
    b) 2, 4
    c) 1, 2, 4
    d) 1, 3, 4
    e) 2, 3, 4

11. Poor renal perfusion, resulting from heart failure, increases fluid volume by:

1. decreasing glomerular filtration of plasma and increasing retention of sodium and water
2. increasing aldosterone secretion which acts on renal tubules to reabsorb sodium and water
3. increasing urination, thereby increasing plasma viscosity and hydrostatic pressure
4. decreasing secretion of renin and subsequent formation of angiotensin

    a) 1, 2
    b) 1, 3
    c) 2, 3, 4
    d) 1, 2, 4
    e) 1, 3, 4

12. Cerebral edema secondary to acute pulmonary edema may manifest itself in:

1. uncooperativeness
2. confusion
3. anxiety
4. apprehension

    a) 1, 2, 3
    b) 1, 2, 4
    c) 1, 3, 4
    d) 2, 3, 4
    e) all of the above

Debriefing

We have all heard that first impressions can be deceiving. Patients who do not appear seriously ill may indeed be quite critical. However, in cases of congestive heart failure, the patient puts all the cards on the table in their facial expressions, breathing pattern, and general appearance. The visible strain in talking, moving, and a general look of exhaustion are most often plainly evident. A drawn and pale face accompanying the audible sounds of fluid bubbling and gurgling with each respiration leaves little doubt that the patient is seriously ill.

Once it is clear that the patient (in this case, Mrs. Atwater) is in distress and that a mismatch in ventilation and perfusion is ongoing, it would be prudent to provide her immediately with a high concentration of oxygen. This is important in order to reduce hypoxemia and its resulting cerebral hypoxia, which may manifest itself as agitation, confusion, or even uncooperativeness on the part of the patient.

The patient in this case was cooperating, but her responses were rambling. In interviewing the patient, it is important not to cut her off too soon. Mrs. Atwater's first concern was not her immediate problem, but the need to relate the absence of her late husband. Patience and empathy at this stage will gain her trust and help to speed the process later on.

Audible congestion in an obese elderly patient is usually accompanied by a long history of similar episodes, because a failing heart is no longer able to keep up an adequate cardiac output and the resulting backup in circulation gives rise to pulmonary edema. In Mrs. Atwater's case, however, the episode of distress is occurring for the first time. What is the underlying cause? Myocardial infarction (MI) should be kept in mind as a real probability throughout the investigation.

We are habituated to thinking that heart attacks involve middle-aged to elderly men complaining of chest pain. In reality, heart attacks are the third leading cause of death, behind lung cancer and breast cancer, among women. While chest pain is one of the most common symptoms associated with myocardial infarction, it is sometimes absent among patients with a history of diabetes. This presentation is termed a silent MI. General malaise and fatigue may be the only symptoms provided.

Mrs. Atwater has two significant predisposing factors often found in the history of patients with cardiovascular disease: diabetes and obesity. In addition, there are a number of stressors that may have contributed to the overall risk of developing an MI. These include the recent death of her husband combined with the family stress of Thanksgiving. There is also stress in eating a large meal as increased myocardial demands are required to meet the rise in metabolic rate. At the same time, there is often an increased sodium intake, which promotes fluid retention and increased circulatory volume, resulting in additional stress to the heart.

The most significant sign in assessing recent history in this case is related to onset. Mrs. Atwater was awakened with dyspnea, which is often described as a feeling of suffocation. Some patients even relate nightmares of drowning or strangulation just prior to waking up. Paroxysmal nocturnal dyspnea is the term given to what is a classic sign of the heart's inability to adequately pump the blood volume it is presented with. As blood waits in the left ventricle to get out, it backs up the system. The result is an increase in pressure throughout the pulmonary vasculature as blood waits to get through. The subsequent increase in hydrostatic pressure in the pulmonary capillaries forces fluid into adjacent alveoli (wet lungs).

Valvular defects (leading to stenosis and regurgitation), chronic systemic hypertension, and myocardial infarction are the most common reasons for heart failure. Since the blood volume entering the left ventricle has not changed, but the ability to clear the volume has, there will consequently be a backup in the system. The backup of blood inevitably extends to the lungs, where high hydrostatic pressures force fluid from the pulmonary vasculature into the alveoli. As the condition worsens, the patient often shows a progression of sleep patterns in which extra pillows are used until the patient is sleeping in an almost sitting position. This orthopneic position allows the fluid accumulating in the alveoli to drain, through the aid of gravity, toward the lung bases, allowing the upper lobes to be relatively clear. The result is a greater ventilation-perfusion ratio in the upright position.

In Mrs. Atwater's situation there were no previous episodes, no history to suggest chronic heart failure of a valvular or hypertensive nature, and no history of previous infarcts. This leaves acute myocardial infarction as a distinct possibility.

Auscultation of heart sounds is a helpful assessment tool. A third heart sound, caused by rapid filling into a non-compliant ventricle during early diastole, and a fourth heart sound occurring late in diastole, when the atria contract into an already full ventricle, are often heard individually or in combination when an MI has occurred. Tachycardia, however, may make distinguishing S.3 and S.4 gallops difficult in the field.

When backup within the vascular system becomes severe, the signs of right-sided heart failure may be seen; however, obesity may make detection of jugular vein distention and other signs difficult.

Although the paramedics were frustrated when they discovered that the small elevator would not accommodate the stretcher, they also discovered an unforeseen benefit in the use of the stair chair. It allowed the legs to be dependent, pooling fluid in the extremities and thus decreasing venous return.

Despite Mrs. Atwater's relief in sitting, the gravity of this situation was brought home when postural vital signs revealed hypotension. Failing cardiac output is an ominous sign, indicating that cardiac contractility is substantially reduced, even when under maximum adrenergic stimulation.

Follow-Up

Mrs. Atwater was assessed in the emergency room and given morphine sulfate, which, besides relieving anxiety, acts as a vasodilator promoting venous pooling and decreasing preload, thus reducing myocardial workload. Additional furosemide (Lasix), a potent diuretic, was given IV to alleviate pulmonary edema. Additional treatment also included nitroglycerin while monitoring blood pressure.

A 12-lead electrocardiogram (ECG) revealed an extensive anterolateral wall myocardial infarct. Mrs. Atwater was transferred to intensive care, having been diagnosed with left-sided congestive heart failure secondary to myocardial infarct. She eventually recovered and was released from hospital to be closely monitored by her family physician.

Fact from Fiction

Women are just as susceptible to the development of atherosclerosis as men. The main difference is that for women before menopause the level of circulating estrogen helps to slow the progress of the disease, while after menopause the risk of atherosclerosis is almost the same as that for men.

Other risk factors indicate that low levels of HDL (high-density lipoproteins) appear to be a more important factor in the development of atherosclerosis than high levels of LDL (low-density lipoproteins). Regular aerobic exercise promotes an increase of HDL, the so called "good" cholesterol. Women with male pattern obesity—gaining weight in the abdomen—will bring an additional risk factor. Upper body obesity predisposes an individual to the development of cardiovascular disease. Most women gain additional weight lower down on the hips (pear vs. apple shaped).

Diabetes, particularly when insulin resistance is the cause, appears to be riskier for women than men. A "silent MI" may be the presentation due to neuropathy that often complicates diabetes.

Smoking is an important risk factor for the development of heart disease, and whereas there has been an overall decline in the number of people smoking, smoking among young women has unfortunately been on the rise. Chemicals from tobacco damage the vascular endothelium, promote vascular spasm, increase platelet aggregation and fibrinogen levels, and increase the overall viscosity of blood. Additionally, tobacco promotes an increased LDL and lower HDL levels. Finally, the increased levels of carbon monoxide within the blood promotes ischemic damage to the endothelium.

Women experiencing a heart attack may have atypical chest pain or may present with dyspnea as the chief complaint.

Answer Key & Rationale

1. b) The congestion referred to in left-sided heart failure describes a fluid shift from the pulmonary vasculature to the air sacs of the lungs. Failure of the left ventricle to adequately pump results in the backup of blood throughout the pulmonary vasculature.

Cor pulmonale refers to right-sided heart failure often seen with emphysema. Right-sided heart failure may also result from valvular defects in the right ventricle or from ischemic coronary disease.

Pulmonary edema develops secondary to left heart failure but is not synonymous with it. Many distinct causes such as near-drowning, pneumonia, and respiratory distress syndrome may all lead to pulmonary edema.

2. c) The most common cause of heart failure is atherosclerosis leading to occlusion of coronary arteries and subsequent ischemia and necrosis of myocardial tissue. This form of heart failure is intrinsic since it occurs within the heart muscle.

Chronic systemic hypertension (essential, the result of renal disease, or the result of other pathology) forces the heart to work harder in order to circulate the blood volume. Constantly high diastolic pressures result in hypertrophy of the heart muscle and subsequently an increase in metabolic and oxygen demands. Over time, the body has increasing difficulty in meeting these demands, and the heart fails.

Aortic stenosis and regurgitation refer to valvular defects, which reflect an inadequate emptying of the ventricle. This mechanical failure is one of improper opening or closing of valves, often the result of scarring associated with a history of rheumatic fever. The ventricle fails to empty adequately, and as a result, pressures rise within the main pumping chamber. The increased pressures extend and stretch the myocardium beyond the optimal range according to Starling's law, weakening contractility and further decreasing cardiac output. Both systemic hypertension and valvular defects are extrinsic to the myocardium.

Anemia, which is also extrinsic, can be a source of heart failure; however, it is less common. The pathology follows a decrease in the oxygen-carrying capacity of blood, resulting in anaerobic metabolism and metabolic acidosis. In response, heart rate and stroke volume increase to meet perfusion demands. Chronic anemia, if severe, will lead to heart stress, cardiomegaly, and eventual failure.

3. d) When the left ventricle is unable to pump effectively and adequately clear its blood volume, the result is an increase in pressure within the chamber. Increases in preload and end diastolic pressure result in a backlog of blood waiting to get in the left ventricle. The result is increased pressure in the left atrium, in the pulmonary vein, and throughout the pulmonary vasculature. The rising hydrostatic pressure forces fluid from the pulmonary capillaries into the alveoli causing congestion and edema.

4. e) Orthopnea is dyspnea that occurs when lying down and may be a sign of the onset of heart failure. Relief is attained when sitting or standing. The onset of heart failure may coincide with the patient's increased desire to sleep in a chair instead of lying in bed. Paroxysmal nocturnal dyspnea occurs when a patient awakens from sleep with dyspnea and a sense of smothering or suffocating. It is a classic sign associated with heart failure. The pink-tinged frothy sputum of acute pulmonary edema, along with wheezing that resembles bronchial asthma, often completes the picture. Postural dyspnea is seen equally in both men and women; the extent of this dyspnea depends on the left ventricle's ability to meet the demand.

During heart failure, chest pain is the most common complaint among men. Palpitations, which usually signal supra-ventricular tachycardia are common to both men and women.

5. d) Acute pulmonary edema develops when the interstitium and alveoli fill with fluid, and can be cardiogenic or non-cardiogenic in origin. In cardiac-related pulmonary edema, pump failure of the left ventricle is the cause. The effect mimics a dam; when the pressure rises high enough, fluid is forced into the lungs. This happens when capillary hydrostatic pressure exceeds colloid osmotic pressure and a fluid shift occurs.

Pulmonary edema, which develops from a non-cardiogenic cause, often does so as the result of increased capillary permeability. This allows fluid containing colloids, which are large molecules, to leak through the capillary membrane into the interstitium and alveoli. Because of the fluid's high colloid osmotic pressure, more fluid tends to be pulled in.

6. a); **7.** c)   Hypoxemia is the result of impaired gas exchange, as alveolar fluid interferes with oxygen transfer across capillary membranes.

Tachypnea arises as the pneumotaxic center is sensitized to a decreasing pH in blood plasma. The respiratory center recognizes the need for more oxygen and increases the rate of breathing.

Crackles and wheezes are the result of air passing through fluid-filled airways during inspiration and are often referred to as cardiac asthma.

Dyspnea is the result of engorged pulmonary vessels compromising lung compliance, making lung expansion more difficult.

Frothy, pinkish sputum is the result of air mixing with protein-rich alveolar fluid. Under pressure, some small pulmonary vessels may rupture, causing red blood cells to leak into the lungs.

Anxiety stems from the feeling of suffocation as the patient tries to catch a breath.

Fever is often associated with causes of pulmonary edema, such as an MI or pneumonia; however, it is not a direct sign.

Dysphagia refers to difficulty swallowing and is not usually directly associated with pulmonary edema.

8. e) There are many non-cardiogenic causes of pulmonary edema. Their pathology often includes a breakdown in the alveolar-capillary membrane. Once the membrane becomes porous, fluid fills the air sacs, compromising ventilation and perfusion.

9. d) High oxygen concentrations will help decrease hypoxemia and allow a greater percentage of oxygen to be available in order to meet metabolic demands. Anxiety, which increases oxygen demand, can be reduced with empathy, reassurance, and proper explanation of all procedures. Fowler positioning allows for maximum descent of the diaphragm and increased lung expansion. The sitting position also allows gravity to drain excess fluid into the base of the lungs, improving the gas exchange in the remaining areas. Elevation of the extremities is counterproductive since it will increase venous return, adding further to the fluid volume in the pulmonary vasculature.

10. c) As cardiac output falls during heart failure, adaptive responses are triggered to help normalize blood pressure and increase cardiac performance. The catecholamines epinephrine and norepinephrine are released to increase heart rate and contractility. The cost is to put added strain on the heart as myocardial demands for oxygen and nutrients are increased. The release of adrenaline also causes peripheral vasoconstriction leading to an increase in the volume of blood returning to the heart. As it is, the failing heart cannot cope with the existing blood volume; therefore, any increase will exacerbate pulmonary edema. Vasoconstriction in renal arterioles along with the release of antidiuretic hormone (ADH) and aldosterone all serve to shut down the kidneys and increase circulating blood volume. In situations of fluid overload, as in congestive heart failure, this adaptive measure is also counterproductive.

11. a) During cardiogenic shock the renal system decreases glomerular filtration, and increases absorption of sodium and water. Angiotensin is created, acting as a powerful vasoconstrictor, decreasing renal perfusion. These actions serve to increase circulating blood volume. Oliguria leading to anuria is a sign of this process.

12. e) Diminished cerebral perfusion results in depression of the CNS and may manifest itself in uncooperativeness, confusion, anxiety, and apprehension, as well as disorientation, somnolence, and coma, if allowed to persist.

CASE STUDY 10

The early spring days were changing snow banks into streams of water that were sluicing down the sidewalks and streets. The driver commented, "On a day like today, it's just as tricky to keep from splashing pedestrians, as to run with lights and siren." Just then, as fate would have it, the call came: a male, forty-eight years old, collapsed—update to follow.

The word "collapsed" is one of those vague terms that leaves all possibilities open. The most useful update is the determination of consciousness, and just as the crew pulled up to the house it was confirmed: patient unconscious.

A visibly distraught middle-aged woman directed the emergency personnel to a detached garage. They entered, leaving the door open, and found the lights on, illuminating a truck with its hood open. On the far side of the truck, a man lay slumped and immobile on the garage floor. While the attending Paramedic initiated a quick primary assessment, the second paramedic assessed the surroundings.

He noted that the patient was not in contact with any electrical equipment, and that the truck was not running. The wife confirmed that the truck had not been running when she found her husband. The gas gauge showed that the tank was half full. Then crew also noticed the distinct smell of something burning. A wood stove stood in the corner, and smoke was billowing out where the stovepipe joined the ceiling. The smoke filled the upper part of the garage; waves of smoke drifted under the fluorescent light fixture above their heads.

The danger was quickly relayed to the attending paramedic, whose observation of the patient revealed no evidence of violence or trauma, nor any external hemorrhaging or burns. The primary assessment, in the process of being completed just as the danger was recognized, revealed a middle-aged male unresponsive to painful stimuli, with palpable carotid and radial pulse, whose respirations showed a pattern similar to Cheyne-Stokes.

The paramedics quickly exited the garage, carrying their patient using the extremities lift. As they left, they silently acknowledged to each other their relief that they had left the garage door open when they first entered. A quick radio call was made to request assistance from the fire department and then they turned their attention to the patient.

Once outside, the patient was provided with 100 percent oxygen and given manual ventilations (bagged) during the periods of apnea, which were lasting between ten and fifteen seconds. The patient was quickly intubated and ventilations were assisted. An IV was started with normal saline and the ECG monitor was attached.

While the stretcher was prepared, further assessment revealed skin pale, pupils dilated bilaterally but reacting, pulse 100 and weak (sinus tachycardia). The stretcher was ready and the patient, Francis Copeland (name provided by wife), was placed semi-prone with head elevated 30 degrees.

Mrs. Copeland was encouraged to come to the hospital, as she also had spent some time in the garage. She rode up front with the driver who learned that Francis was otherwise a healthy non-smoker whose only complaint was occasional early morning back pain. He had previous knee surgery, ligament repair for a sports injury some years earlier, but was not on any medication and had no known allergies.

He went to work in the garage around 10:30 A.M. and she had subsequently gone to tell him lunch was ready around noon. Reflecting on this chain of events, Mrs. Copeland suddenly let out a shriek. She realized that she had left soup boiling on the stove. The EMT notified dispatch that an element could possibly still be on in the house so that the fire department, who had been alerted to the wood stove and smoke hazard, would be notified.

Mr. Copeland remained unresponsive, with periods of apnea and hyperventilation continuing en route. The hospital was informed of a patient with possible severe smoke inhalation or CO poisoning. As the call concluded, Mr. Copeland started to seize. The head was protected and the airway maintained (an oropharyngeal airway had been initially inserted next to the ET tube). The convulsion lasted approximately ninety seconds, whereupon he resumed the Cheyne-Stokes respiratory pattern. Again there was no response to painful stimuli. A radial pulse persisted, although weak and rapid, while the cardiac monitor continued to indicate sinus tachycardia.

Multiple-Choice Questions

1. Carbon monoxide (CO) has:
   1. an orange to brown color
   2. no color
   3. a burnt almond odor
   4. no odor

a) 1, 3
b) 1, 4
c) 2, 3
d) 2, 4
e) none of the above

2. Carbon monoxide is a product of incomplete combustion. Sources include:
1. cigarette smoke
2. automobile exhaust
3. wood fires
4. coal fires

a) 1, 2, 3
b) 1, 3, 4
c) 1, 2, 4
d) 2, 3, 4
e) all of the above

3. Hemoglobin has an affinity for CO that is at least _____ greater than oxygen.

a) two times
b) ten times
c) fifty times
d) one hundred times
e) two hundred times

4. Which of the following statements concerning CO are true?
1. Large amounts of CO are required to produce significant percentages of carboxyhemoglobin.
2. The presence of carboxyhemoglobin strengthens the bond between oxygen and hemoglobin.
3. Since CO is an inhaled toxicant, respiratory acidosis becomes the first clinical sign.
4. CO's toxicity rests in its ability to produce profound hypoxemia leading to hypoxia.

a) 1, 2
b) 2, 4
c) 1, 3
d) 1, 3, 4
e) 2, 3, 4

5. Manifestations of low levels of carbon monoxide poisoning may include:
1. headache
2. tinnitus

3. nausea
4. hallucinations

    a) 2, 4
    b) 1, 3
    c) 1, 2, 3
    d) 2, 3, 4
    e) all of the above

6. Manifestation of low levels of carbon monoxide poisoning may also include:

1. weakness
2. diaphoresis
3. dyspnea
4. dizziness

    a) 1, 2
    b) 2, 3
    c) 1 , 2, 4
    d) 1, 3, 4
    e) all of the above

7. Manifestations of high levels of carbon monoxide poisoning may include:

1. vomiting
2. confusion
3. blurred vision
4. tachycardia

    a) 1, 4
    b) 3, 4
    c) 1, 2, 3
    d) 1, 2, 4
    e) all of the above

8. Manifestations of high levels of carbon monoxide poisoning may also include:

1. cardiac arrhythmias
2. cherry red skin color
3. syncope
4. seizures

    a) 1, 2, 3
    b) 1, 2, 4
    c) 1, 3, 4
    d) 2, 3, 4
    e) all of the above

9. The severity of clinical effects seen in carbon monoxide poisoning depend on the:

1. type of organic material undergoing incomplete combustion
2. concentration of CO in the environment
3. activity level of the victim
4. duration of exposure

    a) 1, 3, 4
    b) 1, 2, 4
    c) 1, 2, 3
    d) 2, 3, 4
    e) all of the above

10. In a normal atmosphere of 21 percent oxygen, half the hemoglobin will be cleared of carbon monoxide in approximately five hours. With the provision of 100 percent oxygen, the time (half life) can be reduced to:

a) 30 minutes
b) 1 hour
c) 2 hours
d) 3 hours
e) 4 hours

11. Hyperbaric oxygen can reduce the half-life of carboxyhemoglobin to:

a) 15 minutes
b) 30 minutes
c) 45 minutes
d) 60 minutes
e) 75 minutes

12. Complications secondary to carbon monoxide toxicity include:

1. pulmonary edema
2. memory impairment
3. myocardial infarction
4. personality deterioration

    a) 1, 4
    b) 1, 2
    c) 2, 3, 4
    d) 1, 2, 3
    e) all of the above

Debriefing

Closed spaces can spell danger. Garages are particularly common sites of carbon monoxide (CO) poisoning. In fact, close to half of all suicides involve carbon monoxide poisoning. The majority of these deaths result from vehicles left running in a closed garage.

For this reason alone, alarm bells should ring when approaching a collapsed individual in a garage. Even if the vehicle is not running, it may be that it has simply run out of gas. Check to see if the keys are in the ignition and note the level of the gas tank.

Another source of carbon monoxide is a barbecue that uses coals or briquettes. To get an early jump on summer barbecuing, some people cook in the garage during cold or inclement weather. Without adequate ventilation, this arrangement carries a significant risk of toxic fumes.

Carbon monoxide itself is odorless and tasteless; in this scenario, however, the smoke from the wood stove carried additional gases of incomplete combustion. The EMT fortunately noticed this burnt smell.

Once the danger of CO poisoning is recognized, the priority becomes the removal of the victim from the environment. The only circumstance that might delay this removal is trauma that indicates a possible spinal injury. If the mechanism of injury (MOI) suggests the possibility of head, neck, or back injury, then the spinal alignment (head to toe in line) should be maintained as the patient is removed. This does not necessitate complete cervical and back immobilization, but simply support for the head and neck, with the body in as straight a line as possible when exiting. Complete immobilization can then be conducted in a safe environment.

Smoke inhalation or CO poisoning, as in the case under discussion, depresses the CNS. Besides a state of unconsciousness, Cheyne-Stokes respirations and seizures indicate the extent of cerebral hypoxia. These clinical features reflect a greater than 50 percent carboxyhemoglobin content.

The most effective method of flushing the system of carbon monoxide is hyperbaric oxygen therapy. As a result, time to delivery of definitive treatment becomes critical. Once the seriousness of the situation is recognized, a load-and-go priority should be considered. The patient should be prepared for transport as soon as the primary patient survey is complete, the chief complaint is recognized, and treatment is initiated in the form of 100 percent oxygen and assisted ventilations during periods of apnea. If a hyperbaric chamber is available at a local hospital, consider transporting there. A quick initial assessment of pulse, respiratory rate, pupils, skin condition, and blood pressure (by palpation) can be conducted at scene; however, if time permits, a complete secondary head-to-toe exam should be conducted, along with additional vitals en route. Even if blood pressure is not measured (as in Mr. Copeland's case), it may be assumed to be at least 80 systolic with the presence of a radial pulse.

Cardiac monitoring was important in Mr. Copeland's scenario, since the degree of tissue hypoxia put him at considerable risk for ventricular fibrillation. Patients suffering carbon monoxide exposure, particularly those with a history of cardiovascular disease, may complain of chest pain consistent with angina or acute myocardial infarction.

Since Mrs. Copeland also spent an undetermined amount of time in the garage, it was prudent that she also be assessed in the emergency room. Pulmonary edema, a complication secondary to smoke inhalation, may not surface until much later. It may take twenty-four to forty-eight hours before irritants from the smoke break down the alveolar-capillary membrane, allowing fluids to seep into the lungs.

Follow-Up

In the emergency room, Mr. Copeland was diagnosed with carbon monoxide poisoning, was continued on 100 percent oxygen therapy and cardiac monitoring while anti-convulsant medication was given to control seizures, along with mannitol and dexamethasone to reduce cerebral edema.

Blood gas values indicated a carboxyhemoglobin level greater than 50 percent. An air ambulance was called to transfer Mr. Copeland to a facility with a hyperbaric oxygen chamber.

Within an hour of arriving in the emergency room, Mr. Copeland had been transported by helicopter and was placed in a hyperbaric chamber at 2 atmospheres of pressure.

Mr. Copeland subsequently regained consciousness, remained free of cardiac anomalies, but was admitted to the hospital where he was monitored closely for neurologic sequelae.

The fire department found that the wood stove had not been used all winter and during the late fall squirrels had nested in the upper portion of the pipe. An inadequate seal where the stovepipe joined the roof led to the release of smoke into the garage. They put out the fire, cleaned the chimney, and rescued the pot from the stove.

Fact from Fiction

Carbon monoxide is one of over 280 separate toxic substances contained in wood smoke. It is the most toxic of the compounds because it displaces oxygen. Hemoglobin, the iron-protein compound which normally carries oxygen in blood, is saturated with carboxyhemoglobin (COHb). The decrease in oxygen-carrying capacity and oxygen release at the tissue level leads to systemic tissue and organ hypoxia. Since hemoglobin stays bound to CO and the remaining oxygen, use of pulse oxymetry for the measurement of oxygen saturation will be unreliable. Remember also, carboxyhemoglobin is bright red and cyanosis, an important sign of widespread hypoxia, may not be evident.

Carboxyhemoglobin is normally less than 2 percent in healthy individuals (higher in urban-city centers with high smog levels and lower in rural-country settings), 5 to 10 percent in cigarette smokers, and may be 20 to 80 percent in instances of CO poisoning, depending on the amount and length of exposure. An important physiological feature of carboxyhemoglobin is a shift in the oxyhemoglobin dissociation curve to the left. The curve describes the relationship between the partial pressure of oxygen in blood and hemoglobin saturation. The adverse effect of a shift in the curve to the left is to impair the release of oxygen at the tissue level. Normally (given a person at rest) at least a quarter of all oxygen getting to the tissues is released to these cells leaving venous blood 75 percent saturated. In the presence of carbon monoxide poisoning, not only is there less oxygen to go around but much of what does get there stays bound to hemoglobin and circulates back into the venous system. The result leaves a profound state tissue hypoxia.

At carboxyhemoglobin levels above 50 percent, death can occur from cerebral hypoxia and cardiac dysrythmias. The elimination of a 50 percent level of COHb at normal room air to a 20 percent acceptable level would take seven hours. Meanwhile, tissue ischemia and organ damage are progressing. If 100 percent oxygen is provided, the time it would take to go from 50 percent to 20 percent is approximately two hours. Given 100 percent oxygen at 2.5 atmospheres (hyperbaric oxygen), the time to 20 percent COHb level from 50 percent would be less than thirty minutes. Given the seriousness of complications and the life-threatening potential of high levels of carboxyhemoglobin it is paramount to start definitive treatment without delay.

Answer Key & Rationale

1. d) Carbon monoxide is an odorless, colorless, and tasteless gas. Elements that may be detected by the senses are separate components of the product of incomplete combustion. Examples include the tar, nicotine, and even cyanide found in cigarette smoke.

2. e) Cigarette smoke, automobile exhaust, wood fires, coal fires, barbecue briquettes, and other forms of incomplete combustion of carbonaceous materials all form the gas carbon monoxide. During exposure, inhalation becomes the route of entry. Interestingly, another source of CO poisoning is methylene chloride (paint stripper): if it is ingested or inhaled, the body converts it to carbon monoxide.

3. e) Hemoglobin will preferentially bind to carbon monoxide. The combining power of CO is between two and three hundred times greater than that of oxygen. This greatly reduces the oxygen-carrying capacity of erythrocytes.

4. b) The presence of carboxyhemoglobin creates stronger bonds between the remaining oxygen and hemoglobin. The result serves only to intensify the existing hypoxia, since the little oxygen that is combined to hemoglobin is not easily released to the tissues.

    The combining influence of carbon monoxide is so great that minute amounts can produce significant percentages of carboxyhemoglobin. Both respiratory and metabolic acidosis are late-stage developments of CO poisoning. Early signs may be slight dyspnea and an intermittent headache.

5. c); **6.** d) Signs and symptoms of moderate to low toxicity levels of carbon monoxide include headache, often throbbing in nature; tinnitus or a roaring sensation in the ears; nausea; weakness or fatigue; dyspnea; and dizziness (vertigo). These symptoms are often associated with carboxyhemoglobin levels of 20 to 40 percent in the blood.

7. e); **8.** e) Signs and symptoms of moderate to high toxicity levels of carbon monoxide include vomiting; confusion or disorientation; visual disturbances such as blurred vision; tachycardia and cardiac arrhythmias; cherry red skin condition (usually a sign of end-stage poisoning); syncope; seizure; and coma. These signs and symptoms are often associated with carboxyhemoglobin levels of 40 to 60 percent in the blood. Levels greater than 60 percent risk fibrillation and cardiac arrest.

9. d) The effects of carbon monoxide are the same no matter what the source and are based on the concentration of CO in the environment and the activity level of the individual at the time of exposure (the more active the individual, the greater the rate and depth of respirations, leading to greater amounts of gas consumed). Obviously, high concentrations over a prolonged period of hard work or exercise will present an increased danger.

    The risk is also high for people who have a prior history of cardiovascular disease; respiratory dysfunction such as chronic asthma, bronchitis or emphysema; and blood dyscrasia such as anemia.

    Workers who are often exposed to carbon monoxide include fire fighters, coal miners, and garage mechanics.

    A fetus is at particular risk from the effects of carbon monoxide since fetal carboxyhemoglobin levels are likely to be 10 to 15 percent greater than maternal levels. Children, as well, probably have an increased susceptibility to CO.

10. b) The half-life of carboxyhemoglobin (the time it takes carboxyhemoglobin levels in the blood to be reduced 50 percent) is approximately five hours in room air (21 percent oxygen); therefore, the provision of 100 percent oxygen, five times the normal amount in room air, can reduce the half-life to approximately one hour.

11. a) A hyperbaric oxygen tank is sometimes referred to as a decompression chamber. It increases both partial pressure and the amount of dissolved oxygen in blood, and can reduce the half-life of carboxyhemoglobin to between ten and fifteen minutes at 2 atmospheres of pressure (one atmosphere is 760 mmHg at sea level; two is 1520 mmHg).

12. e) Complications due to carbon monoxide poisoning include pulmonary edema, particularly with smoke inhalation where pollutants can break down the alveolar-capillary membrane. Since the toxic effects are greatest in tissues with the highest metabolic rates, the heart and nervous system are particularly susceptible. Myocardial infarction, arrhythmias, stroke, and even cardiac arrest are potential complications of CO poisoning. Seizures, as well as mental and personality impairment, are all potential neurological complications of carbon monoxide toxicity.

CASE STUDY 11

There seemed nothing extraordinary about the call the paramedics were given: a routine transfer of an elderly woman who had been in the hospital for a hip replacement. Now, in her second week post-surgery, she was to be taken back to the nursing home. It had been a typically busy day, which meant that the call had been delayed from early morning. Being a low-priority transfer it had been pushed back several times because of incoming emergencies, which meant that it was now late afternoon.

Upon arrival at the hospital nursing station, the ambulance crew was handed the transfer notes. The notes revealed the recent hip surgery (right side) and that their patient Imogene Stone had slight dementia and had recently been diagnosed with Alzheimer's disease. The paramedics found their patient resting on top of the bed, legs crossed, fully dressed with coat and scarf on. Mrs. Stone had been ready since 9:00 A.M. and insisted she was not going to miss her opportunity to "escape," as she put it.

The assessment of Mrs. Stone by the crew was cursory at best. They observed an obese elderly female, notes indicated sixty-nine years of age, who appeared alert and oriented, despite being repetitive with her questions. Her color appeared good and there were no signs of any kind of distress. Vital signs were not completed, with the rationale that it was a low-priority transfer originating in hospital. With physiotherapy Mrs. Stone had been ambulatory with a walker but had not been out of bed all day.

Mrs. Stone was placed in semi-Fowler position on the stretcher and made comfortable. She seemed somewhat anxious but was without complaints. While travelling down the elevator and through the hospital corridors she required constant reassurance that she was being taken to the nursing home and not to the operating room or to have x-rays.

The call continued to be uneventful as the patient was transferred to the ambulance and the journey to the nursing home commenced. The attending paramedic, in chatting with Mrs. Stone, uncovered a fascinating past, which revealed a career as a foreign correspondent. Mrs. Stone had worked and reported from many countries often at times of conflict. Although her stories sometimes repeated, it was clear she had led a remarkable life. It was during one of these stories that Mrs. Stone quite suddenly grabbed her chest and, leaning forward, cried out that she was suffocating.

Her airway appeared clear and she was immediately given a high concentration of oxygen by non-rebreather mask. Mrs. Stone was now complaining of chest pain along with dyspnea and appeared pale and diaphoretic. Vital signs indicated a pulse of 120 full and regular, respirations 32 and regular but gasping in nature, and a blood pressure 132/88. Auscultation of the chest revealed bilateral wheezing. In order to be able to auscultate, the attending paramedic asked her partner to pull over to the side of the road and turn off the engine. At the conclusion of her assessment she asked her partner to join her in the back of the ambulance to help her. The cardiac monitor was attached and showed a supraventricular tachycardia. An IV was quickly inserted. Then the crew proceeded quickly back to the hospital and contacted the emergency department by radio. Information relayed indicated they were arriving with a conscious sixty-nine-year-old female complaining of acute dyspnea and diffuse chest pain.

En route back to the hospital a second set of vital signs was partially completed and revealed a pulse of 128 full and regular; respirations 32 regular and shallow; color indicated peripheral cyanosis (nailbeds); and jugular vein distension was in evidence even with the patient sitting fully upright. As Mrs. Stone was taken into the ER she started a bout of hiccupping, and continued to complain of dyspnea and chest pain along with pain to her right shoulder. In addition, Mrs. Stone seemed quite confused and disoriented.

Multiple-Choice Questions

1. An embolism may exist as:
1. air
2. fat
3. thrombus
4. amniotic fluid
5. talc
6. tumor fragment
   a) 1, 3
   b) 2, 4, 5
   c) 1, 3, 4, 5
   d) 1, 2, 3, 5, 6
   e) all of the above

2. Predisposing factors in the development of a pulmonary embolism often include:
   1. congestive heart failure
   2. long-term immobility
   3. pneumothorax
   4. varicose veins
      a) 1, 2, 4
      b) 2, 3, 4
      c) 1, 2, 3
      d) 1, 3, 4
      e) all of the above

3. Predisposing factors toward the development of a pulmonary embolism often include:
   1. chronic fatigue syndrome
   2. thrombophlebitis
   3. chronic pulmonary disease
   4. recent surgery
      a) 1, 3, 4
      b) 2, 3, 4
      c) 1, 2, 4
      d) 1, 2, 3
      e) all of the above

4. Predisposing factors toward the development of a pulmonary embolism also include:
   1. defibrillation
   2. oral contraceptives
   3. lower extremity fracture
   4. rheumatoid arthritis
      a) 2, 3, 4
      b) 1, 2, 4
      c) 1, 3, 4
      d) 1, 2, 3
      e) all of the above

5. Signs and symptoms produced by pulmonary embolism may include:
   1. hemoptysis
   2. stridor
   3. chest pain
   4. dysphagia
      a) 1, 2
      b) 1, 3
      c) 2, 3, 4

d) 1, 2, 4
e) all of the above

6. Signs and symptoms produced by pulmonary embolism may include:

1. cyanosis
2. tachypnea
3. diaphragmatic breathing
4. bradycardia

 a) 1, 4
 b) 1, 2
 c) 2, 3, 4
 d) 1, 3, 4
 e) all of the above

7. Signs and symptoms produced by pulmonary embolism may include:

1. syncope
2. wheezing
3. splinting
4. hypotension

 a) 1, 3
 b) 2, 3
 c) 1, 3, 4
 d) 1, 2, 4
 e) all of the above

8. Pulmonary embolism can be mistaken for:

1. pneumonia
2. spontaneous pneumothorax
3. acute pericarditis
4. myocardial infarction

 a) 1, 2
 b) 2, 4
 c) 1, 2, 3
 d) 1, 3, 4
 e) all of the above

9. The acid-base imbalance most likely to occur in the initial stages of pulmonary infarction is:

a) decreased PO_2 and respiratory alkalosis
b) increased PO_2 and respiratory acidosis
c) increased PO_2 and respiratory alkalosis
d) decreased PO_2 and respiratory acidosis
e) none of the above

10. Prophylactic therapy for heart patients with a history of atrial fibrillation who are at risk for the development of emboli may include the daily administration of aspirin to:
   a) reduce inflammation
   b) prevent lipid sludge
   c) increase prothrombin time
   d) dissolve small clots
   e) inhibit platelet aggregation

11. Life-threatening complications of pulmonary embolism may include:
   1. pulmonary hemorrhage
   2. pulmonary infarction
   3. pulmonary hypertension
   4. right-sided heart failure
      a) 1, 2, 3
      b) 1, 2, 4
      c) 1, 3, 4
      d) 2, 3, 4
      e) all of the above

12. Treatment of pulmonary embolism in the field should include:
   1. giving ASA (Aspirin) to help break up the blood clot
   2. providing oxygen therapy with a non-rebreathing mask at high concentration
   3. massaging the extremities in order to break up any clots that have formed through venostasis
   4. elevating the legs to promote venous return
      a) 2
      b) 1, 2
      c) 2, 3
      d) 1, 2, 4
      e) 1, 3, 4

Debriefing

Acute dyspnea can arise from many possible causes. A good list to review is the "10 Ps of dyspnea with rapid onset":

pneumonia
pneumothorax
pulmonary constriction (asthma/cystic fibrosis)

peanut (foreign body/anaphylaxis)
pulmonary embolus
pericardial tamponade
pump failure (congestive heart failure)
peak seekers (high altitude)
poisons (toxic inhalants)
psychogenic (hyperventilation)

Pulmonary embolism (PE) can be insidious and difficult to nail down. The best battle plan is to keep a high degree of suspicion when transferring patients who can be identified at particular risk for developing PE.

Deep vein thrombosis from the lower extremities is the source of most thrombi, which find their way to the lungs. Blood clots may, however, also originate in the pelvic veins, upper extremities, and heart chambers.

A thrombus when dislodged, usually due to increased venous pressure or trauma, travels through the venous circulation and enters the right side of the heart continuing on out through the pulmonary artery and into the pulmonary vasculature. The thrombus once it breaks free is called an embolus, and once in the pulmonary circulation it may lodge at the bifurcation of pulmonary arteries or arterioles occluding circulation to a segment, or lobe(s), of the lung. If the embolus is small or there are multiple emboli, the blockage occurs in the pulmonary capillaries, affecting subsegmental vasculature or alveoli.

Once the pulmonary blood flow is obstructed, a ventilation/perfusion (V/Q) mismatch develops. This is where an area of lung is ventilated but not perfused. Dead air space is created, which results in atelectasis and increased pulmonary vascular resistance.

A massive PE by definition obstructs more than 50 percent of the pulmonary vasculature and may well cause cardiac and respiratory failure.

Now that the pathology has been summarized, we can turn to those risk factors that started our discussion. The main triad of risk factors include venous stasis, hypercoagulation, and vascular injury. Venous stasis often occurs when activity is restricted, particularly with patients who are convalescing or on mandatory bed rest. Hypercoagulation is often associated with dehydration, sepsis, age over forty, malignancy, pregnancy, and smoking. Vascular injury in this context refers to catheterization, which increases the risk of thrombus, and surgery, where the problem may not show up until five to ten days post-operative. Additional risk factors include varicose veins, thrombophlebitis, and leg fractures.

Remember that risk factors are cumulative, and in this case our patient, Imogene Stone, was elderly, on restricted activity, and a post-surgical patient, placing her in a high-risk category leading us to maintain an equally high index of suspicion. Other potential contributing factors include her restrictive clothing and the prolonged crossing of her legs, which may have added to the venous stasis. It is also possible that in her protracted wait for the ambulance she may have neglected adequate hydration.

The most common complaint of PE and often the only one is a sudden onset of dyspnea. The patient may seem especially apprehensive or anxious with a sense of impending doom and their fears may well be right on target.

The reason that risk factors play such an important role is that many of the signs and symptoms for PE may be undifferentiated from respiratory problems ranging from asthma to pneumonia, and/or heart ailments ranging from myocardial infarction to acute pericarditis. These signs and symptoms include tachypnea, tachycardia, pleuritic pain, fever, cyanosis, cough, hemoptysis, wheezing, cardiac arrhythmias, diaphoresis, jugular vein distension, and syncope. In addition, cerebral hypoxemia may lead to altered level of consciousness evidenced by confusion and disorientation. As well, a massive PE will lead to hemodynamic changes indicated by hypotension. It is important to note that without ensuring that a baseline set of vital signs is taken (not done in this case), the potential complications that may arise from a seemingly routine transfer can be seriously underestimated. All calls, no matter what their originating priority, require a baseline set of vitals. Vital signs when repeated are important indicators of patient status and direction. They are an essential part of the monitoring process of all patients. In this case lack of time prevented a second blood pressure, which may have revealed a decreasing pulse pressure. Hemodynamic compromise will call for a more aggressive treatment regimen in the ER.

The hiccupping and referred pain to the right shoulder seen in this case indicate that the diaphragmatic pleura is most probably involved. Irritation of the phrenic nerve creates the false message of shoulder pain.

Treatment includes a non-rebreather mask providing 100 percent concentration of oxygen with the patient maintained in a Fowler position (if hemodynamic changes do not contradict). The cardiac rhythm should be monitored for dysrhythmias and recorded. An intravenous line with D_5W or normal saline at TKO should also be established if protocol allows. As well, be prepared to assist with ventilations (BVM) if breathing becomes severely compromised.

A final note in closing this discussion commends the attending paramedic for being interested enough in her patient to have chatted with her en route, which had the fortunate consequence of being able to recognize an immediate change in status. It can be that the only presenting sign of PE is syncope, and if the attendant is engrossed in paperwork or paying little attention to his or her patient, the time delay to recognition and treatment could have dire consequences. Many calls are so-called "routine" transfers, which don't always provide the adrenaline rush of emergency calls; however all calls, no matter what their priority, should be evaluated for potential risk and complications.

Follow-Up

After evaluation in the emergency room a myocardial infarction was ruled out, however blood gases did indicate hypoxemia. Chest x-rays and ventilation/perfusion scan pointed toward an acute pulmonary embolism, which was later confirmed with pulmonary angiography. During the acute phase, 100 percent oxygen concentration was maintained, an intravenous line was started for rehydration, morphine was ordered for pain, and aminophylline, a bronchodilator, was also given.

Anticoagulant therapy with administration of heparin was chosen since thrombolytic therapy with streptokinase or urokinase was contraindicated in view of Mrs. Stone's recent hip surgery. Mrs. Stone was closely monitored for any acute bleeding and checked regularly for partial thromboplastin time (PTT), hemoglobin, and hematocrit levels.

Imogene Stone was released on oral anticoagulants (Warfarin, Coumadin), with physiotherapy and an exercise regimen after three days. She was also encouraged to keep well hydrated.

Fact from Fiction

Pulmonary embolism (PE) carries a very high mortality rate, estimated at 25 percent, with 75 percent of those dying within two hours of onset of symptoms. Early recognition and treatment can reduce the mortality rate to less than 10 percent.

The pathology, which complicates PE, goes well beyond a ventilated but underperfused area of lung tissue. The devastating effects of PE can be seen in the vast majority of cases and not just in instances of massive occlusion and pulmonary infarction (necrosis of the lung parenchyma, which occurs in less than 15 percent of cases). The mechanism which allows PE to be so damaging includes a reflex bronchoconstriction in not just the immediate area of involvement but adjacent areas as well. Bronchoconstriction results from the release of neurohumoral substances, histamine and seratonin. It is considered to be compensatory, an attempt to even out the ventilated and perfused areas of the lungs. The result, however, is to create significant hypoxemia in the area surrounding the occlusion by PE.

In addition, as pulmonary arterial pressures rise because of mechanical obstruction to blood flow, an added workload is placed on the right ventrical which can lead to right-sided heart failure. At the same time a rapid rise in right ventricular pressure can cause a shifting of the ventricular septum toward the left ventricle, impeding filling and subsequent output. Complications arising from a reduction in stroke volume and lower cardiac output include decreased coronary artery perfusion leading to myocardial ischemia and cardiogenic shock.

Recognizing pulmonary embolism in the field is never an easy task, however catching this one in time may make all the difference.

Answer Key & Rationale

1. e) Catheterized patients are most at risk for air embolism. A fat embolus is a potential complication of fractures, particularly long bone (femur) fractures. Thrombi (blood clots) are the most common cause of emboli, with over 50 percent originating in the deep veins (below knee) of the legs. Amniotic fluid can enter the uterine veins creating a serious complication for the expectant or delivering mother. Talc in the form of a precipitate through parenteral administration of medications can create emboli. Tumor fragments may be dislodged, travelling through the venous system, ending up at the heart, and then moving on and lodging in the pulmonary vasculature.

2. a); **3.** b); **4.** d)   Predisposing factors for PE include long-term immobility, chronic pulmonary disease, previous history of PE, congestive heart failure or atrial fibrillation, thrombophlebitis, varicose veins, cardiac arrest or defibrillation, recent surgery, advanced age, pregnancy, extremity fractures, burns, obesity, malignancy, oral contraceptives particularly in combination with smoking, coagulation disorders, sepsis (especially IV drug abuse), and dehydration.

5. b); **6.** b); **7.** e)   Signs and symptoms for PE include a classic triad of hemoptysis, pleuritic chest pain (acute on inspiration), and dyspnea. However, this triad is seen in less than 30 percent of patients. Chest pain and dyspnea are the most commonly reported symptoms. Additionally there may exist a cough, apprehension, anxiety, syncope, tachypnea, fever, rales/crackles, wheezing, pleural friction rub, distended neck veins (JVD), dysrhythmias, chest splinting, and signs of circulatory collapse (tachycardia, diaphoresis, hypotension, and hypoxia with cyanosis).

8. e) Pneumonia and myocardial infarction often present with similar signs and symptoms to PE making differentiation difficult. Both acute pericarditis and a spontaneous pneumothorax list signs and symptoms similar to PE. The best evidence for differentiation in the field lies in eliciting a thorough history. Predisposing factors for the development of PE may provide some of the most important clues.

9. a) The shunting of blood in the pulmonary vasculature following a PE and the resulting V/Q mismatch leads to a state of hypoxemia which is reflected in a decreased PO_2. Tachypnea in combination with anxiety and apprehension will lead to a state of hypocapnia. The decreased PCO_2 in the lungs results in respiratory alkalosis. As the state of hypoxemia persists, tissue hypoxia will follow, and the resultant anaerobic metabolism will lead to a state of metabolic acidosis.

10. e) Enteric (coated) acetylsalicylic acid (ASA or aspirin) acts as an anticoagulant (blood thinner) by inhibiting platelet aggregation. The clumping together of platelets is an essential part of the clotting process.

11. e) Without prompt intervention in acute PE, life-threatening complications include pulmonary hemorrhage; pulmonary infarct as the area of ischemia leads to necrosis; pulmonary hypertension with the shunting of blood; acute cor pulmonale with heart failure; dysrhythmias including ventricular fibrillation; and the development of subsequent pulmonary emboli.

12. a) Patients with PE may present with orthopnea and should be seated upright to allow for maximum lung expansion. In a massive PE the hemodynamic changes leading to shock may preclude the Fowler position. A 100 percent oxygen concentration should be delivered in the presence of a PE even if the patient has a history of COPD (Chronic Obstructive Pulmonary Disease). Remember to include an explanation of all procedures along with plenty of reassurance in order to help alleviate anxiety, which in itself will increase oxygen demand.

Extremities should never be massaged as any inflamed areas may dislodge emboli, which will further compromise the patient's condition. If the source of the PE was from deep vein thrombosis (DVT) then elevation of the extremities will potentiate additional emboli. ASA does not assist in the break-up of clots.

Once a diagnosis has been made in the ER, anticoagulant therapy with heparin is generally considered to be the treatment of choice. Although controversial, thrombolytic therapy to dissolve existing clots is another option. Heparin does not act to dissolve the thrombus; its role is to keep it from enlarging and to prevent further thrombi from forming while the body's natural fibrinolytic mechanism dissolves the existing clot.

CASE STUDY 12

The call came through at the end of a long, hot day. It was the first really warm weekend of the newly arrived summer and the crew was looking forward to the end of its twelve-hour shift. It was 6:45 in the early evening, fifteen minutes before the end of the shift, when the call came, a standby at a working fire. The ambulance crew arrived on scene just minutes behind the fire department. It was enough time, however, for the fire department to have assisted a young man by providing him with thermal blankets and portable oxygen.

The crew approached the patient, who was seated on the front lawn, and quickly assumed responsibility from the fire department. The attending paramedic set about ensuring that airway, breathing, and circulation were adequate. It did not appear that there was evidence of inhalation injury, no singed nasal hairs or burns to the face or neck, and the patient, who stated his name was William Gorman, spoke without hoarseness. The airway was clear and a quick assessment of breathing revealed tachypnea, without dyspnea or any obvious wheezing. The radial pulse was weak and barely palpable but the EMT knew it at least reflected a BP of 80 systolic. There was no evidence of gross bleeding, however, there were obvious second and third degree burns to both the front chest and abdomen and covering half the back, as well as the right arm and upper front thigh of the right leg.

Sterile water was poured in copious amounts over the burns, while the other paramedic went about gathering information from the fire department and setting up the stretcher. Sterile burn sheets were laid out on the stretcher.

The clothes that could easily be cut off were removed. As the crew worked they were unable to escape the smell of burnt flesh, which had a sobering effect on all. The work was completed efficiently and with few words. William was quickly lifted onto the stretcher with the help of six fire fighters (two holding the stretcher in place). He was positioned supine with legs elevated. Sterile dry burn dressings were loosely applied over the burns. A cardiac monitor was placed on the patient in a slightly modified position with the positive lead on the left thigh and the negative lead placed on the top of the right shoulder. The patient was wrapped in the sterile burn sheets and the oxygen administration of 100 percent concentration by non-rebreathing mask was continued. An IV with lactated Ringer's solution was inserted in William's left (unburned) arm and run wide open.

The information gathered revealed that William had set up the barbecue, turned the propane on, and gotten distracted by a phone call. Not realizing he had already turned the gas on, he ignited a flame and was about to turn it on when the explosion occurred. The gas had already been running for several minutes. The ensuing explosion resulted in his clothes being set on fire. He had rolled on the ground in order to put out the flames.

Throughout the experience William had been complaining of pain, especially to his right arm and leg where the skin was showing signs of blistering. As preparations for transport were ongoing he seemed to be getting quite anxious and somewhat confused, wanting repeated explanations as to what happened. Since he appeared shocky and had a declining LOC, he did not meet the criteria for implementing the pain management protocol.

En route additional information revealed William to be thirty-four and weighing approximately 175 lbs (80 kg). A set of vitals revealed: LOC—oriented to name only; pulse 128 weak and regular; cardiac rhythm was sinus tachycardia; respirations 34 shallow and regular; blood pressure 98 by palpation; pupils slightly dilated at 6 mm, equal and reactive; skin showing peripheral cyanosis to lips and nail beds along with delayed capillary refill.

The local burn center was contacted and advised about William's injuries and status. An estimate of the percentage of burn (40 percent second and third degree), vital signs, and time of arrival was also provided.

On arrival at the burn center, while the cardiac rate remained unchanged, the blood pressure now showed 88 by palpation and William responded verbally to painful stimuli by groaning only. As he was being wheeled into the center the cardiac monitor indicated intermittent premature ventricular complexes (PVCs).

Multiple-Choice Questions

1. In differentiating between second- and third-degree burns, the third-degree burn presents with:
   1. white tissue
   2. red tissue
   3. black tissue
   4. analgesia
   5. blisters
   6. hypo to hyperalgesia

      a) 1, 3, 4
      b) 3, 5, 6

      c)   1, 2, 5
      d)   2, 3, 6
      e)   1, 2, 4

2. Determine the percentage of body surface area (BSA) as expressed by the rule of nines for a burn, that involves the abdomen and the front of both legs in an adult patient.

      a)   18 percent
      b)   27 percent
      c)   36 percent
      d)   45 percent
      e)   54 percent

3. Important factors to take into consideration, which may increase the seriousness of a burn:

   1.   location; e.g. face, hands, feet, genitalia
   2.   configuration; e.g. circumferential burns
   3.   history of chronic disease; e.g. atherosclerosis, diabetes
   4.   concurrent injuries; e.g. fractures, internal injuries
   5.   patient age; e.g. children and elderly
   6.   pulmonary injury; e.g. smoke inhalation

      a)   1, 2, 4, 6
      b)   1, 3, 4, 5
      c)   2, 3, 4, 5, 6
      d)   1, 2, 3, 5, 6
      e)   all of the above

4. A major full thickness thermal burn will produce a pathophysiology, which can include:

   1.   central nervous system impairment leading to Cheyne-Stokes respirations
   2.   altered membrane permeability with loss of electrolytes
   3.   burn wound exudate leading to evaporative fluid loss
   4.   release of histamines leading to increased capillary permeability

      a)   1, 2, 3
      b)   2, 3, 4
      c)   1, 2, 4
      d)   1, 3, 4
      e)   all of the above

5. Pathophysiologic factors seen in major thermal burns include:

   1.   carbonization of cells leading to cell lysis
   2.   vasodilation leading to increased capillary permeability
   3.   coagulation leading to a massive pulmonary embolus

4. disruption of cellular and humoral immunity leading to increased risk of infection
    a) 1, 2, 4
    b) 1, 3, 4
    c) 2, 3, 4
    d) 1, 2, 3
    e) all of the above

6. Hypovolemia and decreased cardiac output as seen in major thermal burns results from:
1. anaemia following red blood cell destruction
2. increased capillary permeability
3. peripheral vasodilation
4. evaporative fluid loss
    a) 1, 2, 3
    b) 2, 3, 4
    c) 1, 2, 4
    d) 1, 3, 4
    e) all of the above

7. Swelling from edema associated with burn shock:
1. occurs primarily in the area of the burn and is not systemic
2. is associated with the release of prostaglandins, thromboxanes, histamines, and serotonin
3. may compromise distal circulation in areas of circumferential burns
4. may lead to mechanical airway obstruction, necessitating tracheal intubation
    a) 1, 2, 3
    b) 1, 2, 4
    c) 1, 3, 4
    d) 2, 3, 4
    e) all of the above

8. The main constituents of the solution Ringer's lactate are:
1. glucose
2. sodium
3. potassium
4. protein
5. bicarbonate
6. chloride
    a) 1, 2, 4, 5
    b) 3, 4, 5, 6
    c) 2, 3, 5, 6
    d) 1, 3, 5, 6
    e) 1, 2, 4, 6

9. In estimating the burn percentage in a small child the EMT should take into account that the:

1. head comprises a larger percentage than an adult
2. trunk (abdomen, chest, and back) comprises a smaller percentage than an adult
3. legs comprise a larger percentage than an adult
4. arms comprise a smaller percentage than an adult

  a) 1, 2
  b) 1, 3
  c) 2, 4
  d) 1, 3, 4
  e) 2, 3, 4

10. Complications that may arise during management of extensive thermal full thickness burns include:

1. hypovolemia
2. myoglobinuria
3. septicemia
4. hypothermia

  a) 1, 2, 3
  b) 2, 3, 4
  c) 1, 2, 4
  d) 1, 3, 4
  e) all of the above

11. If the percentage of burn is 40 percent and the weight of the patient is 175 lbs (80 kg), the fluid replacement during the first hour should be approximately:

  a) 200 ml
  b) 400 ml
  c) 600 ml
  d) 800 ml
  e) 1000 ml

12. Management goals in the initial treatment of thermal burns are to:

1. pour water or a solution over the burns in order to completely stop the burning process
2. maintain aseptic technique at all times in order to reduce the risk of subsequent infection

3. recognize that the integumentary system in part determines personal identity, heightening the need for empathetic delivery of care
4. guard against hypovolemia, decreased cardiac output, and shock by providing adequate fluid replacement

    a) 1, 2, 4
    b) 1, 3, 4
    c) 1, 2, 3
    d) 2, 3, 4
    e) all of the above

Debriefing

Thermal burns provide one of the most difficult challenges to emergency medical personnel. The challenge rests not only with the medical management but also with the psychological stress inherent in these calls. Burns can literally tear away the fabric of who we are. Our identities are inextricably married to how we look. Just as our hearts go out to young children when involved in trauma and illness, we can easily identify and empathize with burn victims. In order for emergency personnel to cope with this type of trauma it is important to have a forum for discussing the feelings and sentiments these calls engender. Critical incident stress debriefings are an important part of acknowledging that we are all human and help to reaffirm the caring side of our nature, which has directed us into the health-care field in the first place.

Burns touch a raw nerve with emergency personnel; it may be the personal identification (since most are accidental it is easy to think *there but for the grace of God go I*), the moving sight of the burn victim, or the smell of burnt flesh, which is never forgotten. As a result it is essential to concentrate and focus on the efficient and effective management of the burn patient to quickly minimize the life-threatening risks of airway/breathing problems and circulatory problems leading to hypovolemic shock, as well as the subsequent risk of infection leading to septic shock.

Thermal burn management includes the obvious removal of the patient from the source followed by stopping any active burn (if within fifteen to twenty minutes) through wetting the burn with normal saline or distilled water if available. Any water source is ultimately acceptable so that stopping burn progression is the main priority and aseptic technique a secondary concern. The process of continuous cooling of burns should be restricted to a maximum of one minute, since there is a strong risk of hypothermia associated with cooling for prolonged periods of time. Airway assessment includes noting singed nasal hairs, hoarseness, stridor, and facial burns, which are all indications of inhalation burns. Note also that circumferential burns of the neck could produce edema and circulatory constriction producing airway obstruction. Circumferential burns are rarely a problem on the scene; however, they could pose a major complication during subsequent interfacility transport. Smoke inhalation and subsequent pulmonary edema along with the risk of hypovolemic shock should all be taken into account and 100 percent oxygen should be given by non-rebreather. The absence of wheezing or dyspnea does not always mean that all is well, since hemoptysis and rales/crackles may not show up until a day or two later. The application of burn dressings and sterile blankets, maintaining warmth, and positioning for shock round out the management for the basic provider.

The use of dry vs. wet dressings is still undergoing some debate so check local protocols. The basic advantage to wet (moistened—damp not soaked) is the alleviation of heat and pain. They are also less likely to stick to burns, causing less damage on removal. Dry dressings have the advantage of minimizing infection and hypothermia.

Fluid infusion is also a major treatment modality and if allowable should be started without delay, running at least one line (large-bore 16 gauge) wide open with lactated Ringer's, an isotonic electrolyte solution. Avoid starting the line through burned tissue. Total fluid given should be noted and reported as both fluid intake and output will need to be closely regulated in the burn unit.

Remember to provide ongoing reassurance, as this is a very scary experience, both physically and emotionally traumatic for the patient.

When dealing with burns, use aseptic technique whenever possible to guard against the potential for infection. Besides the obvious route for bacteria to enter, the physical stress of coping with major thermal burns weakens the body's immune system, opening the door to opportunistic infections.

On a very practical note, because of the edema, rings and other constrictive jewelry should be removed from the patient and placed for safe keeping. The heart should be monitored for dysrhythmias, which can arise from a decreased cardiac output, electrolyte imbalance and/or acidosis. Vital signs are closely monitored to determine evidence of hypovolemic shock.

Shock can set in quite rapidly in patients with major thermal burns, the earliest signs being restlessness and confusion as was seen with William. Postural or orthostatic vital signs can also be an early indicator of the progression toward hypovolemic shock. The indicator is an elevated pulse and narrowed pulse pressure (difference between systolic and diastolic) when the patient goes from supine to sitting or standing. The patient might also complain of lightheadedness or syncope.

Transporting without delay is also an important part of field management, and completion of a comprehensive secondary assessment may have to be conducted en route. Mechanisms of injury (e.g., hazards in a burning building) should be taken into consideration. There always exists the possibility of spinal trauma and appropriate measures should be taken if it can't be ruled out. Treat the patient under trauma protocol and major burns as "load and go" following primary assessment and intervention, keeping on-scene time to under ten minutes if possible. Taking blood pressures by palpation can also save a little time in that it can be done even with sirens blaring. The systolic pressure recorded by palpation is likely to be 10 mm Hg below the actual systolic if auscultated.

Most often with burns, there will likely be a lot of emergency personnel, especially fire crew around to help. Make use of their presence, get them to help where possible, since an efficient team effort takes the burden off any single rescuer and provides everyone with a sense of accomplishment particularly important in the face of such devastating injuries.

Follow-Up

William was diagnosed with thermal burns, 25 percent third-degree and 15 percent second-degree, as well as hypovolemic shock. He was aggressively treated with fluid replacement therapy (lactated Ringer's). Endotracheal intubation was performed and blood was drawn for complete blood count, electrolytes, glucose, blood urea nitrogen, creatinine, arterial blood gases, and type and cross match. Clothing stuck to the patient was removed after being soaked in saline. Devitalized tissue was debrided, taking care not to break any blisters. Topical antimicrobial and antibiotic agents were used with non-stick dressings. The PVCs seen on arrival dissipated once the blood pressure was brought under control. Later on in order to assist in breathing, escharotomy of the chest was performed. A tetanus prophylaxis was also ordered.

The hospital stay was not uneventful for William. At the end of his first week he battled a massive infection, which lead to septic shock. William survived his ordeal, and with skin grafts, pain medication (morphine pump), extensive use of the hyperbaric chamber (to promote healing), and much psychological support, he was eventually released to home care. In addition William underwent extensive physiotherapy to prevent contractures.

The theory behind hyperbaric oxygen therapy is that the oxygen demand of injured tissue is at its highest when it is least available. The only effective method of significantly increasing the oxygen content of blood is to dissolve greater amounts in plasma. When atmospheric pressure is doubled the amount of dissolved oxygen in the plasma can be boosted to fifteen times its usual level, pumping more oxygen into injured tissue, which promotes faster healing. In addition, the elevated pressure of oxygen reduces blood flow by as much as 20 percent, which decreases capillary blood pressure. There are still megalevels of oxygen in the blood because of the large amount dissolved in the plasma, and the reduced blood pressure reverses the tendency for fluid to accumulate in injured tissue, which helps to impede swelling.

Fact from Fiction

The skin is the largest organ in the body, weighing in at 20 percent of total body weight; it not only encloses the body, but interacts functionally with all body systems. A major burn will have a profound effect on all organ systems. Starting in the burned area and eventually cascading into all aspects of homeostasis, a burned patient will experience disruption and alteration in immune response, electrolyte balance, metabolism, thermoregulation, as well as functioning of the cardiovascular, respiratory, renal, and GI systems.

The stress that a burn exerts on the body drives catecholamine levels up; elevates cortisol, glucagon, and insulin levels; and increases the metabolic rate with ongoing glycogenolysis (breakdown of glycogen stores to glucose). Hypermetabolism, which results, keeps and resets the thermal regulatory set point at a much higher rate. Typical core body temperature may be 101°F (38.5°C).

Higher than normal metabolic rates will significantly increase the heart rate, often above 120 per minute, as well as oxygen consumption to 150 percent of normal. As oxygen needs increase the respiratory rate rises to meet the demand. For every 2°F (1°C) increase in basal metabolic rate, respirations increase by four breaths a minute. Additional fluid loss results as respiratory rates rise.

Hypermetabolism, hyperthermia, and hyperglycemia can all be present in the systemic stress response to burns. Even the GI system is not impervious to the effects of burn stress. A very common stress ulcer of the intestinal wall among burn patients is known as Curling's ulcer.

Stress also brings about translocation of micro-organisms, a consequence of selective sympathetic vasoconstriction and a decrease in opsonins (normally occurring substance that enhances phagocytosis). Bacterial translocation in the presence of a weakened immune system makes infection almost inevitable.

Despite the adverse response, stress actually plays an important role in the physiologic drive to regain health and homeostasis in a burn patient. Recovery from major burns, however, is long and involved, and complications are the rule rather than the exception.

Answer Key & Rationale

1. a) The white or carbonized black tissues that present in third-degree or full thickness burns indicates a depth of burn below the dermis. The result is that nerve destruction leaves the site pain free. Third-degree burns also destroy the tissue's regenerative properties and healing is difficult unless the area is small or skin grafting is possible.

The classic sign of a second-degree or partial thickness burn is that of blisters.

2. b) In the "rule of nines" for adults the head represents 9 percent, the abdomen and chest (trunk) 18 percent, the back 18 percent, the arms 9 percent each, and the legs 18 percent each. A burn involving the abdomen which is half the trunk (half of 18 percent) and the front of both legs (half 18 percent × 2) results in 9 percent plus 18 percent and equals 27 percent burn surface area (BSA). Note—the palm of the patient's hand represents approximately 1 percent BSA.

3. e) Major burns are third-degree that comprise a BSA of 10 percent or greater, or second-degree of 30 percent or more. Burns are also considered critical if they involve the face, hands, feet, and genitalia.

Vascular disease, especially diabetes and heart disease, can complicate fluid replacement, and pulmonary disease can cause a more severe reaction to smoke inhalation.

Other injuries sustained at the time of the burn can contribute to hypovolemic shock.

Children have less total fluid volumes in their vascular system and are at greater risk for shock. Their immune system is not as fully developed and as such they are at a higher risk for complications.

The elderly lose the elasticity of their blood vessels and their glands are not as capable as they once were of releasing compensatory amounts of hormones to battle the stress of shock. These two factors along with a depressed immune system put them at greater risk for the complications of burns.

4. b) The carbonization of cells that take place in thermal burns results in the disruption of cellular membranes releasing potassium and vasoactive substances including histamines. The electrolyte imbalance can lead to cardiac arrhythmias while the release of histamines and other vasoactive substances will lead to fluid loss from the vascular system. Contributing to hypovolemia in thermal burns is the evaporative loss of fluid from burn wound exudate.

Although the central nervous system may be depressed due to cerebral hypoxia, Cheyne-Stokes respirations are not often seen unless associated with head injuries sustained during the fire.

5. a) As stated in question 4, the carbonization of cells will break down their membranes and spill the contents. The heat and vasoactive substances will vasodilate capillaries, increasing their permeability, allowing fluid to shift out into the interstitial space. The immune system will become depressed as a result of thermal burns. Both cellular (neutrophils and eosinophils participating in phagocytosis) and humoral (lymphocytes participating in the production of antibodies) immunity is disrupted, increasing the potential for infection and sepsis.

While coagulation may take place with thermal burns and pulmonary emboli is always a concern, a large pulmonary embolus is not an often seen complication.

6. b) Increased capillary permeability results in a porous or leaky vascular bed with fluid volume shifting out into the interstitial space. Vasodilation of peripheral blood vessels results in increased capillary permeability and a pooling of blood in the periphery. Burn wound exudate results in a loss of fluid through evaporation. All of these factors result in a decreased vascular fluid volume and a decreased venous return, resulting in a decreased cardiac output, reduced blood pressure, and poor perfusion.

Anemia, which results from the destruction of erythrocytes (red blood cells), will contribute to hypoxemia and hypoxia; however it does not contribute to a decreased fluid volume.

7. d) Through the release of vasoactive substances (prostaglandins, thromboxanes, histamines, and serotonin) the increased capillary permeability allows fluid to move out of the vascular system, causing edema that is systemic.

Circumferential burns may constrict the circulation and escharotomy may need to be performed in order to release pressure. Massive edema and swelling around the neck may cause a partial or total airway obstruction necessitating endotracheal intubation.

8. c) Lactated Ringer's solution is a crystalloid that does not contain protein. Colloid solutions contain varying percentages of protein, sugar, and starch molecules. Colloids may promote edema in patients with increased capillary permeability. These protein-rich fluids may leak from the capillaries into the interstitial compartment, decreasing intravascular volume.

Lactated Ringer's is an electrolyte solution containing sodium, potassium, chloride, and bicarbonate.

9. b) The head of a small child is about double the surface area of that of an adult. The trunk (chest, abdomen, and back) and arms are equal in the percentage surface area to those of an adult. The legs of a child comprise a relatively smaller percentage of total surface area than that of an adult. Note also that the pediatric patient has a high surface area to body weight ratio, which means the fluid reserves for burns are low.

10. e) Hypovolemia results from an inability of damaged blood vessels to contain plasma. A shift of plasma proteins (albumin) and fluids into the burn tissue will reduce the blood's ability, via osmosis, to draw fluids from the uninjured tissues. Concurrent increased capillary permeability and peripheral vasodilation contribute to a decreased venous return.

Myoglobinuria and haemoglobinuria resulting from destruction of muscle tissue and red blood cells respectively may be seen in thermal burns. Free myoglobin in the vascular system may clog renal tubules and decrease renal perfusion.

The breakdown in the immune system can lead to infections and septicemia. Remember with thermal burns there is open communication to the outside and a direct route for bacteria to enter the body.

The skin senses temperature and provides for a normothermic environment. The loss of skin integrity leaves the body susceptible to hypothermia. Rapid cooling of the burn area will also contribute to a generalized hypothermia.

11. b) A commonly used calculation for fluid replacement in a burn patient is known as the Baxter formula. The patient's weight in kilograms is multiplied by the total burn surface area (BSA) and multiplied by a constant (4 mls) providing the total fluid volume to be given over twenty-four hours. Half the total fluid volume will be given over the first eight hours. The amount to be given during the first hour for a patient weighing 80 kilograms with a 40 percent BSA is as follows:

(80 kg × 40 percent × 4 ml) / 2 = 6,400 ml in 8 hours

6,400 ml/8 hours = 600 ml/hr

The intravenous administration set appropriate to rapid infusion will deliver 10 gtt/ml. Since the amount of fluid to be infused in one minute is 600/60 = 10, then the drip should be set at 10×10 = 100 gtt/min. The large amount of fluid required will likely necessitate two IVs running at 50 gtt/min. each.

12. e) The burning process may be still active for a short while after contact with the fire or thermal energy. This burning process is short-lived, usually lasting no longer than fifteen minutes. Pouring water over burns should take the above into account as well as the risk of hypothermia if there is a large burn surface area to deal with.

Aseptic technique should be maintained at all times when dealing with burn patients to reduce the risk of infection. Wearing gloves, using sterile dressings and sheets, along with distilled water or saline will help reduce the risk of infection.

Providing reassurance and maintaining a caring and professional attitude is an essential part of the management of all calls and deserves special emphasis when dealing with the trauma, both physical and psychological, of burns.

Hypovolemic shock is the immediate life-threatening complication of major thermal burns and fluid therapy (electrolyte solution) is essential to stem a decrease in cardiac output and subsequent fall in blood pressure.

CASE STUDY 13

The rain, which was falling heavily, seemed to let up for a few moments as the call was given out by dispatch. The information was brief: an unconscious three-year-old. No other clues were forthcoming other than the address, which was just on the outskirts of the city.

With a little time to the destination, the crew reviewed the most likely possibilities for which a young child can be found unconscious. Trauma seemed obvious—kids fall and bang their heads—so they made a mental note to consider spinal immobilization. Drowning was mentioned but the day was overcast and raining so the possibility that kids would be around a pool seemed remote. The final thought they had with trauma rested on the possibility of children playing with improperly stored firearms. Neither of the paramedics wanted to reflect on this one for long. They then switched their attention to medical causes, discussing respiratory causes that could lead to unconsciousness. Airway obstruction seemed an obvious possibility along with the possibility of an acute asthma attack. Epiglottitis also came to mind as an upper airway obstruction, however the age seemed a little young. Another medical possibility discussed was accidental poisoning and overdose, with the medics making a mental note to call poison control if a substance could be identified.

As the discussion was drawing to a close, with the consideration of febrile seizures seeming a real possibility while congenital cardiac anomalies seemed somewhat more remote, the crew arrived on the scene.

They were met by a frantic mom, who gave absolutely no information that made any sense. They were directed through the open garage door at the back of which they found the child.

The attending paramedic was able to quickly determine the following: airway clear; breathing adequate; no signs of obvious trauma; patient responsive to touch with incoherent words; constricted pupils; pulse bradycardic; diaphoresis; and incontinence.

While patient assessment was in progress the second paramedic was able to establish that three-year-old Amber was playing in the garage with her older sister Andrea when she found a bag of powder which they thought was flour like mom had in the kitchen. Amber had reached in and managed to ingest some and started almost immediately to cry. Andrea, who fortunately had not touched the bag, ran to get her mom.

There were chemical residues on Amber's face, hands, and clothing. The powder was gently brushed off and contaminated clothing removed.

A garden hose was utilized to quickly flush the hands. The chemical residue on the mouth proved a little more difficult to remove and Amber was starting to have some airway difficulty with a lot of secretions developing. Suction was employed followed by a 100 percent concentration of oxygen by non-rebreather. Concern over a bradycardic apical rate led to the hook-up of the cardiac monitor, which showed a sinus bradycardia.

While the second paramedic took note of the chemical names on the bag (chlorthion and parathion) and called the poison information center, he also noted that Andrea was crying and complaining of a stomach ache. While waiting for a response from Poison Control, he took Andrea aside and said she might feel more comfortable sitting down and distracted her by helping her put her shoes on. He let Andrea know it wasn't her fault and commended her for getting help so quickly. Miraculously, her tummy ache went away.

The paramedics quickly inserted an IV of normal saline. Atropine 0.02 mg/kg was administered IV in an attempt to relieve the bronchorrhea. Amber was quickly prepared for transport with a more thorough set of vital signs to be taken en route.

Poison Control informed the EMTs that they were dealing with an organophosphate poisoning and that they were to transport stat, watching for respiratory depression and hypotension. En route respiration dropped to less than ten a minute and Amber was manually ventilated between respirations. The emergency room was informed of their young arrival and by the time they entered the resuscitation room Amber was starting to seize.

Multiple-Choice Questions

1. The uses of organophosphate chemicals include:
   1. insecticides
   2. pesticides
   3. herbicides
   4. chemical warfare agents
      a) 1, 2, 3
      b) 1, 3, 4
      c) 1, 2, 4
      d) 2, 3, 4
      e) all of the above

2. Which of the following statements concerning the actions of organophosphates are true?

1. Inactivation of cholinesterase occurs at the synaptic junction.
2. They cause decreased levels of the neurotransmitter acetylcholine.
3. Paralysis of nerve impulse transmission occurs across the myoneural
junctions.
4. As acetylcholine fails to accumulate in the parasympathetic nervous
system, the organs affected are understimulated.

   a) 2, 4
   b) 1, 3
   c) 1, 2, 4
   d) 1, 2, 3
   e) all of the above

3. Poisoning by organophosphates can occur through which of the following
routes:

1. gastrointestinal
2. respiratory
3. ocular
4. dermal

   a) 1, 2, 4
   b) 1, 3, 4
   c) 2, 3, 4
   d) 1, 2, 3
   e) all of the above

4. A mnemonic SLUDGE lists a number of signs and symptoms typical of
organophosphate poisoning. These include:

1. septicemia
2. lacrimation
3. uremia
4. diaphoresis
5. gastrointestinal distress
6. emesis

   a) 2, 5, 6
   b) 1, 4, 6
   c) 2, 3, 4, 5
   d) 1, 3, 4, 6
   e) 1, 2, 3, 5

5. Signs and symptoms reflecting the effects of organophosphate poisoning
on the cardiovascular system include:

1. bradycardia
2. atrial fibrillation

3. A-V blocks
4. hypotension
   a) 1, 2, 4
   b) 1, 2, 3
   c) 1, 3, 4
   d) 2, 3, 4
   e) all of the above

6. Signs and symptoms reflecting the effects of organophosphate poisoning on the respiratory system include:

1. hyperventilation
2. dyspnea
3. stridor
4. rales/crackles
   a) 1, 3
   b) 2, 3
   c) 2, 4
   d) 1, 2, 4
   e) 1, 3, 4

7. Signs and symptoms reflecting the effects of organophosphate poisoning on the CNS include:

1. slurred speech
2. paresis
3. miosis
4. seizures
   a) 1, 4
   b) 2, 4
   c) 1, 2, 3
   d) 2, 3, 4
   e) all of the above

8. Life-threatening complications related to organophosphate poisoning, are usually the result of:

1. hepatic failure
2. pulmonary edema
3. respiratory muscle paralysis
4. hypoglycemia
5. hypotension
   a) 1, 3, 4
   b) 2, 3, 5
   c) 1, 2, 4, 5
   d) 1, 3, 4, 5
   e) all of the above

9. Immediate or delayed ascending paralysis starting in the lower extremities may occur with organophosphate poisoning. This most closely resembles which of the following neuromuscular disorders:

a) myasthenia gravis
b) muscular dystrophy
c) multiple sclerosis
d) Guillain-Barre syndrome
e) amyotrophic lateral sclerosis

10. Which of the following statements concerning atropine sulfate are correct?
  1. It is a potent sympatholytic agent.
  2. It is used in the management of symptomatic bradycardia.
  3. It blocks acetylcholine receptors.
  4. It has both a positive chronotropic and inotropic effect.

    a) 2, 3
    b) 1, 3
    c) 2, 4
    d) 1, 2, 4
    e) 1, 3, 4

11. The effects of atropine sulfate in the treatment of organophosphate poisoning include:
  1. mydriasis
  2. tachycardia
  3. tachypnea
  4. excessive salivation

    a) 1, 3, 4
    b) 1, 2, 4
    c) 1, 2, 3
    d) 2, 3, 4
    e) all of the above

12. Priority management concerns in caring for a patient with organophosphate poisoning include:
  1. transport stat, leaving decontamination of the patient to ER personnel
  2. control airway aggressively through suctioning as needed
  3. closely monitor for cardiac dysrhythmia and hypotension
  4. anticipate CNS depression and seizures

    a) 1, 2, 3
    b) 1, 2, 4
    c) 1, 3, 4
    d) 2, 3, 4
    e) all of the above

Debriefing

Organophosphate compounds are a group of chemicals that have a highly unstable chemical structure and can disintegrate within a few days. For this reason they are widely used as household insects sprays, and in agricultural applications such as insecticides, pesticides, and herbicides. Because of the frequency of use, organophosphates and carbamates (a somewhat less toxic form), poisonings occur in relatively high numbers.

Organophosphates are among the most toxic chemicals currently in use. They were also used in the development of military nerve agents (such as sarin and soman) during World War II, and have recently surfaced as a terrorist weapon.

The main effect of organophosphates is to inhibit acetylcholinesterase, the enzyme that degrades acetylcholine at the neuromuscular junction. Acetylcholine is a cholinergic neurotransmitter. When acetylcholinesterase is inhibited, acetylcholine accumulates at the synapses, and a cholinergic "overdrive" occurs, resulting in the signs and symptoms characteristic of organophosphate poisoning.

When little information is available from dispatch, the receiving crew would do well to review the different possibilities as this crew did, mainly to avoid getting tunnel vision and jumping to conclusions. Amber, who had just turned three, was at that inquisitive age and without fear. The rain meant that the kids were playing indoors, however the garage containing accessible pesticides was definitely not the appropriate playground.

The first order of business on arrival is to remove the cause, which is creating an ongoing hazard. Brushing powdered chemicals off the patient should proceed without delay, taking care never to blow the residue off as a cloud of particles may find their way into the face and eyes of the attendant. Flushing should be liberally conducted with copious amounts of fluid. Contaminated clothing may never completely rid itself of residue, even after many washings, and so should be discarded.

Most localities have a regional poison control center, which can help determine the substance involved, as well as provide management tips. Of course, the first simplest step is to check the label on the container—often, it will contain all of the information necessary to initiate treatment. As always airway and respiratory management are both priorities but of special concern in the case of organophosphate poisoning, since the development of excessive salivation along with respiratory paralysis and pulmonary edema means that airway and respiratory complications may well become life threatening.

EMTs deal with life-threatening calls on a daily basis; however, for a young child like Andrea, who was just a couple of years older than her sister, this was quite a traumatic experience. The way in which the non-attending EMT was able to pay attention to the older sister's needs, will go a long way toward helping her deal with the tragic nature of an event like this no matter what the outcome.

Follow-Up

In the emergency room Amber was confirmed to have organophosphate poisoning. Her airway was managed with endotracheal intubation. Atropine Sulfate 0.05 mg/kg repeated at five-minute intervals was administered, which managed to control the seizures without the use of atavan or diazepam. Paradoxime chloride was also given to counter the effects of organophosphate poisoning (a parasympatholytic agent that inhibits the effects of acetylcholine). Protopam chloride acts to degrade acetylcholine by reactivating the enzyme acetylcholinesterase.

Amber was able to recover, and, considering the toxicity of the chemical agents she was exposed to, she was a very lucky three-year-old.

Fact from Fiction

More than three quarters of all pediatric poisonings occur in children under the age of five. The vast majority of poisonings in this age group are simply accidents. If, however, a small child who is not capable of exploring is poisoned, then look for the possibility of error, child abuse, or the malintentions of an older sibling. It is important to keep an open mind and report accurately all findings, but don't waste time looking for someone to blame. There are probably more than enough feelings of guilt to go around if a child has been involved in accidental poisoning. Remember that your patient is best served by identifying the agent, which is not always an easy task, and initiating appropriate treatment.

If identification of the agent is not possible, then a toxidrome should be established. Based on physical assessment, a picture of related findings, which are characteristic of various classes of poisons, make up the toxidrome.

The cholinergic toxidrome is based on clinical features that relate to parasympathetic stimulation: pinpoint pupils; bradycardia; hypothermia; increased salivation and bronchial secretions; diaphoresis; vomiting and diarrhea; and seizures. Since other toxidromes may share similar findings (the opioid toxidrome, for example, has pinpoint pupils, hypothermia, and bradycardia), a differential diagnosis must rely on a thorough examination of all assessment findings.

The possibilities for accidental poisonings are almost endless, so getting to know some common and well-established toxidromes can prove helpful. Also of use is a critical thinking approach that considers significant clinical features with a view to creating a list of those substances that can produce the symptoms. Seizures, for example, can result from antidepressants, beta-blockers, cocaine, insulin, and certain insecticides among others. At the same time, potential causes of pinpoint pupils could include opioids, alcohol, and certain insecticides. By cross-referencing the common possible causative agents with patient presentation, a most likely candidate may be found.

Answer Key & Rationale

1. e) Organophosphates are widely used as insecticides, pesticides, and herbicides, which means that agricultural workers are most commonly exposed. Because organophosphates are ubiquitous, children are often exposed, resulting in accidental poisoning. They are used as well in flea and tick collars for pets. These substances are so toxic, they are also chemically related to the warfare agents soman, sarin, and tabun.

2. b) Acetylcholine (Ach) is the most widely distributed neurotransmitter, being found in both the peripheral and central nervous system. It is stored in vesicles in the nerve terminal until released into the synapse. Once in the synapse, Ach chemically combines with receptors to produce the desired reaction and is subsequently destroyed by the enzyme acetylcholinesterase.

The organophosphate radical binds with acetylcholinesterase, inactivating it, which allows Ach to accumulate at the myoneural junctions and inhibits the effects of acetylcholinesterase, causing an over stimulation of the parasympathetic system. After first enhanced nerve impulses, there follows paralysis, which may lead to respiratory paralysis, shock, and cardiac arrest.

3. e) Organophosphates can be found as liquids, dusts, wettable powders, concentrates, and aerosols with a garlic-type odor. Routes of exposure include ingestion, inhalation, eye contact, and skin absorption.

4. a) The classic SLUDGE syndrome contains a number of flu-type symptoms: Salivation, Lacrimation, Urination, Defecation, Gastrointestinal pain, and Emesis.

Diaphoresis would be a valid sign for organophosphate poisoning, however it is not part of the mnemonic.

5. c) Overstimulation of the parasympathetic system on the cardiovascular system can lead to bradycardia, ventricular arrhythmias, atrio-ventricular blocks (conduction is slowed through the A-V node), and hypotension secondary to decreased cardiac output.

6. c) The effects of organophosphate poisoning on the respiratory system include dyspnea, along with tightness in the chest (bronchoconstriction), acute pulmonary edema producing rales/crackles, and respiratory paralysis and failure.

7. e) Effects of organophosphate poisoning on the CNS system can include CNS depression, anxiety, headache, dizziness, weakness, loss of muscle coordination, muscle fasciculations, disorientation, confusion, drowsiness, slurred speech, seizures, constricted pupils, and coma.

8. b) The major threats to life with organophosphate poisoning usually involve respiratory failure caused by chemically mediated pulmonary edema, respiratory paralysis, and hypotension following bradycardia.

9. d) Guillain-Barre syndrome is an idiopathic peripheral polyneuritis. Symmetric weakness and paralysis may develop starting in the extremities and ascending to the trunk.

Myasthenia gravis involves muscular weakness especially in the face and throat as a result of a deficiency of acetylcholine.

Muscular dystrophy is a group of genetically transmitted diseases characterized by progressive atrophy of skeletal muscles.

Multiple sclerosis is a progressive disease involving demyelination of nerve fibers of the brain and spinal cord. Symptoms include paresthesia and paresis.

Amyotrophic lateral sclerosis is a degenerative disease of the motor neurons. The disease is manifested through a chronic and progressive muscular atrophy.

10. a) Atropine sulfate is a potent parasympatholytic agent which produces its action by blocking the effects of acetylcholine. It is used in the management of hemodynamically significant bradycardias, particularly the various heart blocks. Although it has positive chronotropic (heart rate) properties, it has little or no inotropic (contraction strength) effect.

11. c) Atropine sulfate will dilate pupils, increase respiratory rates, and in the presence of organophosphate poisoning, should increase the heart rate to at least 120. Additional actions include relaxation of the bronchioles, urinary retention, and decreased motility of the gastrointestinal tract. Once the drug takes effect the patient should stop the excessive salivation.

12. e) In order to decrease the risk of exposure, decontamination should be carried out without delay. Removing the patient from the source, removing contaminated clothing, brushing off residue and flushing with copious amounts of fluid are all management priorities.

Airway management may include ongoing suctioning as excessive salivation can create airway compromise. This should be followed by a 100 percent concentration of oxygen by non-rebreather and a closely monitored respiratory rate. Additional ventilations should be manually provided if the rate falls below 10 per minute and/or the depth of ventilations is inadequate.

Cardiac monitoring should be in place since bradycardia may be present and there can also be a risk of ventricular fibrillation.

In severe cases of organophosphate poisoning CNS depression can potentiate seizures, which will add to the growing state of hypoxia.

All of the foregoing are important concerns and priorities in the management of the patient with organophosphate poisoning, however it is also important to look for any associated trauma, which may go unnoticed.

CASE STUDY 14

The hotline crashed through the two and a half hours of sleep they managed to gain since returning from their last flight. It was just after 4:30 A.M., still dark out, and dispatch was pre-alerting the flight paramedic and pilots of a possible scene response on a major four-lane highway. Within minutes the call was confirmed and the aircraft was ordered to launch. The information provided was that a bus had collided with a tractor-trailer, with multiple patients involved.

The pilots had already started the Sikorski S-76 helicopter with the pre-alert and were discussing the flight route and landing they would be making. The sun was due up at 5:25 A.M. and judging the distance to scene and the 400 km ground speed of the helicopter, it meant they would be making the landing just before sunrise.

As the scene came into view they circled once before landing. The bus was crushed from the front and appeared to have rammed into the back end of the eighteen-wheeler. There were two ambulances (one just leaving the scene), two fire trucks, and about a half-dozen police cars, this later group having blocked out a landing site on the highway.

The flight paramedic had been communicating with the ambulance ground crew and had been informed that two individuals were still trapped near the front of the bus, but were close to being extricated. One of the persons trapped was considered to be in critical condition. In consultation with the pilots it was decided to shut down just one of the two jet engines and keep the blades going. The "hot loading" would allow for a few precious minutes to be saved.

Arriving at the bus the flight paramedic was briefed on the patient and injuries. Franklin Davis, a twenty-six-year-old male, was conscious and oriented, complaining of severe dyspnea. He had contusions on the right side of his chest and an initial set of vitals gave a pulse 96 strong and regular, respirations 24 and labored, blood pressure 114/82, pupils 5 mm equal and reactive, skin cool, pale, and diaphoretic. In addition, no breath sounds were auscultated on the right side.

The driver of the bus had been fatally injured. Franklin had been seated in the second row and had seats in front of him jammed back, pinning his legs. Pelvis and legs were as yet unexamined. A precautionary C-collar had been placed on Franklin and it was not long before the seats in front were removed by the fire department and he could be laid down on a long spineboard. An IV of Ringer's lactate was started and an assessment of the extremities revealed an obvious deformity of the left lower leg, exposure showed a compound tibia/fibula fracture. The leg was quickly immobilized and with Franklin secured to the fracture board and provided with a 100 percent concentration of oxygen by non-rebreather, he was taken off the bus and loaded into the helicopter.

Within seconds they had lifted off with an estimated time of arrival (ETA) of 18 minutes to the trauma center. Because of the potential chest injuries, the flight paramedic requested an altitude ceiling as low as possible, and the pilots maintained an altitude of no greater than 1,500 feet.

On board Franklin was experiencing increasing dyspnea. Further assessment revealed: a pulse of 118 which weakened and almost disappeared with inspiration; respirations were unchanged except for the increased dyspnea; blood pressure 106/78; pupils unchanged; skin now showed cyanosis to lips and mucous membranes; Franklin, who had been extremely anxious on scene asking where he was and what was going on, now had to be repeatedly roused to respond; there appeared to be a tracheal shift to the left side and there appeared subcutaneous emphysema (air leaking into tissues), which could be palpated just below the right clavicle; he was also coughing up a frothy red-streaked sputum; and the oxygen saturation monitor which had initially shown 94 percent was now indicating 85 percent.

The paramedic contacted the trauma center, relayed the latest vital signs including the probability that a tension pneumothorax was developing. Permission was given to perform needle decompression (needle thoracotomy) to relieve pressure. To decompress the pleura the approach taken was to palpate the second intercostal space in the mid-clavicular line and insert a two-inch (12 gauge) over-the-needle catheter just above the third rib at a 90-degree angle. The needle was advanced until air escaped, then the catheter was advanced and the needle removed. The catheter was then secured in place and a one-way valve was created by cutting the finger off an examination glove, rinsing it thoroughly with water, attaching it to the catheter, and making a small hole in the distal end. Relief from dyspnea appeared almost immediately as the S-76 was completing its final approach for landing. Once again the patient was unloaded "hot" and transferred to the care of the trauma team.

Multiple-Choice Questions

1. Blunt chest injuries may include:

1. ruptured pancreas
2. ruptured diaphragm
3. flail chest
4. myocardial contusion
5. hemothorax

   a) 1, 2, 4
   b) 1, 3, 5
   c) 1, 3, 4, 5
   d) 2, 3, 4, 5
   e) all of the above

2. Thoracic trauma may present with:

1. paradoxical chest movement
2. diaphragmatic breathing
3. jugular vein distension
4. subcutaneous emphysema

   a) 1, 2, 3
   b) 1, 2, 4
   c) 1, 3, 4
   d) 2, 3, 4
   e) all of the above

3. Indications of a flail chest may include:

1. diminished breath sounds on the affected side
2. the contraction of the diaphragm during expiration
3. the unstable chest wall is pushed inward during inspiration
4. crepitus elicited on palpation

   a) 1, 2, 3
   b) 1, 2, 4
   c) 1, 3, 4
   d) 2, 3, 4
   e) all of the above

4. Signs and symptoms of a tension pneumothorax include:

1. cyanosis
2. tracheal deviation
3. increasing dyspnea

4. bradycardia
   a) 1, 2, 3
   b) 1, 2, 4
   c) 1, 3, 4
   d) 2, 3, 4
   e) all of the above

5. Rib fractures causing pulmonary contusion often result in:
   1. hyperventilation
   2. hemoptysis
   3. hypoxia
   4. dyspnea
      a) 1, 2, 3
      b) 1, 2, 4
      c) 1, 3, 4
      d) 2, 3, 4
      e) all of the above

6. The most common cause of shock following chest trauma is:
   a) pneumothorax
   b) flail chest
   c) myocardial contusion
   d) pulmonary contusion
   e) hemothorax

7. A tension pneumothorax leading to a mediastinal shift may present with which of the following clinical signs?
   1. paradoxical pulse
   2. jugular vein distension
   3. dysrhythmias
   4. decreased pulse pressure
      a) 1, 2, 3
      b) 1, 2, 4
      c) 1, 3, 4
      d) 2, 3, 4
      e) all of the above

8. Indications of a deteriorating condition in the presence of chest trauma include:
   1. stridor
   2. guarding
   3. altered LOC
   4. inability to talk
      a) 1, 2, 3
      b) 1, 2, 4
      c) 1, 3, 4
      d) 2, 3, 4
      e) all of the above

9. The acid-base imbalance that develops following traumatic chest trauma is most likely to be associated with:
   1. hypoxia
   2. hypoxemia
   3. hypocapnea
   4. hypopnea
      a) 1, 2, 3
      b) 1, 2, 4
      c) 1, 3, 4
      d) 2, 3, 4
      e) all of the above

10. The pathophysiology resulting in a tension pneumothorax can include:
    1. penetrating chest wall or closed puncture of the lung by a fractured rib
    2. air entering the pleural space from within the lung or from the outside, creating a one-way valve effect
    3. accumulating pressure causes partial or total lung collapse with mediastinal shift
    4. the heart, great vessels, and contralateral lung are compressed and pushed to the unaffected side, decreasing cardiac output
       a) 1, 2, 3
       b) 1, 2, 4
       c) 1, 3, 4
       d) 2, 3, 4
       e) all of the above

11. Life-threatening complications associated with chest trauma include:
1. esophageal varices
2. ruptured aorta
3. pericardial tamponade
4. tracheobronchial tears
    a) 1, 2, 3
    b) 1, 2, 4
    c) 1, 3, 4
    d) 2, 3, 4
    e) all of the above

12. Beck's triad, the cardinal features indicative of cardiac tamponade, include
1. cyanosis
2. jugular vein distension
3. chest pain
4. decreased blood pressure
5. muffled heart sounds
    a) 1, 2, 4
    b) 2, 3, 5
    c) 1, 3, 5
    d) 2, 4, 5
    e) 1, 3, 4

Debriefing

Chest injuries can create some of the most urgent life-threatening situations. We only have to look at the organs enclosed in the thorax, the lungs, trachea, heart, great vessels, superior and inferior vena cava, and aorta to understand the significance of just how potentially serious trauma to the chest can be.

It is important to consider the mechanism of injury and carry a high index of suspicion since injuries to the chest are the most frequently missed injuries in the first hour of care.

Rib fractures are the most common chest injuries. They often occur as a result of falls among the elderly, which may produce secondary complications such as atelectasis and pneumonia. Another special group that deserves consideration when rib fractures occur is children. Because a child's ribs are much more elastic, they do not frequently fracture, however this only increases the risk of missing underlying thoracic injuries.

Fractures of the lower ribs may include intra-abdominal injuries particularly to the spleen and liver, two highly vascular organs. Multiple rib fracture of two or more adjacent ribs or a detached sternum allowing for incongruous chest wall movement indicates a flail chest. The result is paradoxical chest movement which allows for the flail section to be drawn in as the diaphragm descends. The forces resulting in a flail chest will almost always mean that there will be associated trauma to underlying structures.

A closed or simple pneumothorax as seen in this case causes a ventilation perfusion mismatch. The fractured rib(s) has caused a loss of negative pressure in the intrapleural space resulting in partial or total lung collapse. The main clinical features are sudden onset of chest pain and dyspnea, absent or diminished breath sounds on the affected side, and hyperresonance on percussion.

The development of a tension pneumothorax is a life-threatening condition. With each inspiration pressure increases in the thoracic cavity as more and more air seeps into the pleural space. The result is not only a collapse of the affected lung but also a push of the mediastinum toward the unaffected side (mediastinal shift). The pressure on the heart and greater blood vessels will result in a reduction in cardiac output as both venous return and cardiac filling are reduced. Pressure on the unaffected lung will also reduce perfusion and compromise ventilation. The clinical features include increasing dyspnea, tracheal deviation toward the unaffected side, jugular vein distension (JVD); decreased blood pressure, and cyanosis. There may also be air leaking into the subcutaneous tissues (subcutaneous emphysema) around the neck and upper chest. In addition, as the pressure tamponades the heart, there may be a decrease in pulse pressure during inspiration when the pressure is greatest. This manifests as a reduction in volume when a pulse, carotid or radial, is palpated. The pulse may actually disappear during inspiration and is called a paradoxical pulse (pulsus paradoxicus). The systolic blood pressure will also fall during the period of inspiration.

Concurrently there may also be the development of a hemothorax. A laceration to the lung allows for blood to collect in the intrapleural space. The lung is a very vascular organ and the accumulation of greater than 1500 ml of blood is considered a massive hemothorax. The clinical manifestations are the signs of hypovolemic shock.

One important consideration in transporting by air a patient with a tension pneumothorax is to limit the altitude, since any trapped air will increase in volume as atmospheric pressure decreases. An altitude of 1500 feet should pose little threat to the expansion of these gases.

A definite ventilation-perfusion imbalance develops in the presence of a pneumothorax, and it will lead to hypoxemia and hypoxia. A pulse oximeter measuring a patient's arterial oxygen saturation will be able to denote any change in tissue perfusion. A significant decrease in oxygen saturation will be a sign of the patient's deteriorating condition.

Follow-Up

In the trauma center Franklin was diagnosed with multiple systems trauma. Injuries included rib fractures leading to a tension pneumothorax and a compound tibia/fibula fracture. A chest tube (under water seal drainage) was inserted to re-establish patency within the lungs and he was closely monitored for any increase in pleural pressure. It was estimated that Franklin had suffered a 70 percent collapse of his right lung and the nature of the tear required surgical repair.

Orthopedic consult was obtained for the leg fracture. There was fortunately no other organ damage and he was eventually able to make a full recovery.

Fact from Fiction

Evaluating chest trauma requires a sound knowledge of both important landmarks and the anatomical structure of the thorax. The chest or thorax encases the lungs with bone, cartilage, and muscle. Respiration is maintained mainly through the actions of both the intercostals and diaphragmatic muscles.

The lungs are contained in the right and left pleural cavities separated by the mediastinum. Each lung has a major fissure (the oblique), which divides upper and lower portions. In addition, the right has another horizontal fissure in the upper portion at the level of the fifth rib in the axilla and fourth rib anteriorly. Each lung rises anteriorly (to the apex) about 4 cm above the first rib into the base of the neck. Posteriorly, the lower border extends down on inspiration to about T12 and rises upward on expiration to T9.

The bronchi, which channel air into the lungs, separate from the trachea into a left and right branch. The right mainstem bronchus is wider and straighter than the left, which accounts for a greater incidence of aspiration into the right lung. Endotracheal tubes, if extended too far, will inflate the right lung only.

Describing the location of findings is best based on the following commonly used landmarks. A good starting point is the suprasternal notch, a depression easily palpable at the base of the neck and just above the manubrium. The ribs are counted starting at manubriosternal junction (angle of Louis) where the second rib joins the sternum. The first rib lies above the clavicle and is not palpable. The intercostal space corresponds to the rib immediately above it.

Anteriorly, the separation of the left upper lobe (LUL) from the left lower lobe (LLL) occurs at the sixth rib in the mid-clavicular line. The sixth rib is also the location for right lower lobe (RLL) and right middle lobe (RML) separation. The location of the fourth rib finds the horizontal fissure between the right upper lobe (RUL) and RML. Posteriorly, the spinous process of T3 separates both RUL from RLL and LUL from LLL. C7 is the first spinous process to be felt with T1 just below.

Landmarking is also aided by referencing the nipple line, and various vertical lines both anterior and posterior including right and left mid-clavicular, right and left anterior axillary, mid-axillary and posterior axillary lines, vertebral line, and the right and left scapular lines. Terms such as medial (toward the inside), lateral (toward the outside), proximal (toward the center), and distal (away from the center) should also be used.

Describing the location of findings using appropriate anatomical landmarks and medical terminology generates accuracy and authenticity in both oral and written reporting.

Answer Key & Rationale

1. d) Blunt trauma to the chest can result in the following injuries: ruptured diaphragm, flail chest, myocardial contusion, hemothorax as well as pneumothorax, pulmonary contusion, ruptured aorta, torn trachea or bronchi, rib fractures, and lacerated liver or spleen.

2. e) Paradoxical chest movement occurs when a flail segment of the chest wall caves in during inspiration. This asymmetrical chest movement is often associated with multiple rib fractures and pneumothorax.

Diaphragmatic breathing refers to abdominal breathing, which in the presence trauma usually means a ruptured diaphragm. The thorax no longer rises and falls with the contraction of the diaphragmatic muscle.

Jugular vein distension (JVD) may be seen in the presence of a tension pneumothorax or pericardial tamponade. Pressure on the mediastinum and heart force a decrease in venous return and stroke volume reducing cardiac output. A backup of blood in the system can be seen as blood engorges the jugular veins, noticeable even when the patient is in a semi-sitting or sitting position.

Subcutaneous emphysema, which may be seen with a pneumothorax, refers to air leading out and accumulating just under the surface of the skin around the neck and upper chest.

3. c) Multiple rib fractures may cause a flail chest where a loss of chest wall integrity prevents adequate lung inflation. The flail segment moves in when the diaphragm contracts during inspiration and bulges outward on expiration. Crepitus (the grating sound of bone against bone) may be noticed on palpation of the rib fractures.

4. a) Increasing dyspnea, tracheal deviation toward the unaffected side, and cyanosis are classic signs for the development of a tension pneumothorax.

Additional signs of shock may also be present, such as diaphoresis, tachycardia, decreased blood pressure, dilated pupils, and agitation. Absent breath sounds and jugular vein distension are also associated with a tension pneumothorax.

5. d) Pulmonary contusion, the result of blunt trauma bruising the lung, can give rise to: a cough with hemoptysis (blood-tinged frothy sputum); dyspnea, particularly exacerbated by deep inspiration in the presence of rib fractures; signs and symptoms of hypoxemia; and splinted (shallow and guarded) respirations which may lead to hypoventilation. The signs and symptoms of a pulmonary contusion may be slow to develop (one to four hours) and can lead to the patient's becoming hypoxic.

6. e) Massive hemothorax is the most common cause of shock following chest trauma. A flail chest with underlying chest injury, pneumothorax, myocardial contusion (leading to arrhythmias and pericardial tamponade), and pulmonary contusion may all lead to shock. The lung is an extremely vascular organ with each side of the thorax capable of holding up to 30 percent of the patient's blood volume.

7. e) A tension pneumothorax is progressive and as pressure builds it compromises the circulatory system. Pressure on the superior and inferior vena cava decreases venous return while pressure on the heart decreases stroke volume. Intrathoracic pressure is at its greatest during inspiration, which accounts for a weak or absent pulse (paradoxical pulse) during this phase of the respiratory cycle. As blood backs up, waiting to enter the right side of the heart, there is engorgement of the jugular veins (JVD). With a reduction in venous return and a decreased stroke volume (blood ejected with each beat of the heart) there will be a decreased cardiac output and a subsequent decrease in pulse pressure. Without adequate perfusion the myocardium will show signs of irritability manifested by dysrhythmias.

8. c) Stridor is a high-pitched sound occurring as air passes through a narrowed larynx. An inability to talk seen in conjunction with chest trauma may indicate increased edema in the upper airway. An altered level of consciousness, confusion, or disorientation may be the result of cerebral hypoxia secondary to a ventilation-perfusion mismatch in the presence of chest trauma.

Guarding is a protective response to pain and may be seen with any rib fracture. In addition splinting, the voluntary limiting of movement, is also a common sign of rib fractures.

9. b) Without adequate ventilatory chest excursion and with decreased lung perfusion following chest trauma, hypoxemia will develop and lead to hypoxia resulting in metabolic acidosis. The decreased tidal volume, the result of splinting or a pneumothorax, will lead to the retention of carbon dioxide (hypercapnia) and a subsequent respiratory acidosis.

10. e) In a tension pneumothorax resulting from a penetrating chest wound (knife, gun shot) or puncture by a fractured rib (blunt trauma), the wound permits air to enter the pleural space, and as a one-way valve is created, a progressive build-up of pressure occurs. As pressure increases, more of the affected lung collapses; and as air continues to accumulate in the pleural space, there is pressure placed on the unaffected lung and the mediastinum. The pressure pinches the inferior and superior vena cava, restricting blood flow to the heart (reduced venous return). The pressure on the mediastinum starts to impinge the functioning of the heart, reducing stroke volume and cardiac output leading to shock.

11. d) The patient with a ruptured aorta rarely survives long enough to reach the emergency department where definitive care can be provided. Pericardial tamponade caused by lacerated pericardium or ruptured coronary artery results in constriction of the heart, reducing cardiac output, and leads to hemodynamic deterioration. Disruption of the tracheobronchial tree carries a high mortality rate within the first hour. The tear most commonly occurs near the bifurcation of the mainstem bronchus, one inch from the carina.

Life-threatening complications associated with chest trauma also include: tension pneumothorax, massive hemothorax, flail chest, diaphragmatic rupture, myocardial contusion with dysrythmias, and traumatic asphyxia, the result of massive crush injury to the chest.

Esophageal varices is a medical problem resulting in distension and rupture of esophageal veins secondary to portal hypertension and often associated with cirrhosis of the liver. Once bleeding occurs it can be life-threatening.

12. d) Beck's triad includes: jugular vein distension as the superior vena cava is pinched and blood backs up in the neck veins; decreased blood pressure and pulse pressure (leading to paradoxical pulse) as outside pressure decreases diastolic filling which reduces stroke volume and cardiac output; muffled or distant heart sounds as fluid fills the pericardial sac.

Additional signs of cardiac tamponade include cyanosis, tachycardia, chest pain, and a deteriorating level of consciousness.

CASE STUDY 15

The ambulance crew was microwaving popcorn. They were at base and had just finished checking off their vehicle. It was game seven of the Stanley Cup hockey finals, and the second period was just getting underway when the call came: fifty-six-year-old male with chest pain. A mental image of a slightly obese man with a history of smoking leading a somewhat sedentary lifestyle was conjured up by the paramedics, then quickly dismissed since they had both experienced young, seemingly fit men with myocardial infarctions (MIs).

Though it is best never to assume or prejudge, the reality in this case was not too dissimilar from the initial mental image created. Joseph Therion was at home in his favorite easy chair watching the game when he started experiencing tightness in his chest. He had finished dinner and was relaxing with his second beer when the pain started. He had suffered a heart attack six months ago and was on propranolol (beta blocker) and nitroglycerin.

Mr. Therion had been experiencing chest "discomfort" as he called it, off and on for the past two days and was getting relief from the nitro pills. This evening he had already taken three sublingual nitro pills without any relief. Despite his pain he had not wanted his wife to call 911 but she had insisted.

The hockey game was still in progress on the TV and Mr. Therion wanted it left on. The medics were both big hockey fans and under any other circumstances would have agreed.

Additional history revealed that Mr. Therion, who had smoked for thirty years, had quit smoking after his initial heart attack. He had recently just resumed work driving a tractor-trailer. He stated he hadn't done anything out of his normal routine today, and that he normally had a couple of beers in the evening after dinner.

Physical assessment revealed an overweight male, diaphoretic, pale, with obvious dyspnea (he had to pause to speak between breaths). Auscultation of his heart revealed an extra heart sound occurring just after the second, his pulse was 66 strong and regular, blood pressure was 112/70, respirations revealed tachypnea, and he was fully oriented.

While reluctant to have all this fuss made over him, Mr. Therion allowed the EMTs to place him on 100 percent concentration of oxygen via a non-rebreather mask and to be placed on the cardiac monitor which did not show any ST segment elevation (lead II) but did reveal what appeared to be a first-degree heart block with a regularly prolonged P-R interval. The date on the nitroglycerin bottle had not expired, and the name on the bottle indicated that medication had been prescribed to him. The paramedics immediately inserted an IV with normal saline.

Mr. Therion fitted the protocol for administration of nitroglycerin. His blood pressure was over 100 systolic and his pulse, despite the delay in conduction between the SA and AV node, was greater than 60. With his permission a .4 mg dose of sublingual nitroglycerin spray was given.

The tightness in the chest Mr. Therion had complained about had been ongoing for the past hour without abating and was radiating up into his jaw. Mr. Therion also fit the protocol for ASA treatment. There were no contraindications: no history of active GI bleeding; no history of clotting disorders; no history of adverse reaction to ASA if known asthmatic; no history of asthma; and finally no recent (within twenty-four hours) history of CVA or head injury. As such, with Mr. Therion's permission, he was given two 80 mg tablets of chewable ASA.

While preparations were made for transport, a follow-up blood pressure revealed a systolic of 108, and a pulse of 58. The nitro spray had not provided the desired pain relief, however a second dose was contraindicated since the pulse had now dropped below 60.

After more than a little convincing, Mr. Therion finally agreed to be taken to the hospital, and while being transferred into the ambulance he stated he was feeling extremely nauseous. This latest complaint sounded an alarm in the mind of the attending EMT. An emesis basin was provided and the suction equipment was readied just in case. En route Mr. Therion was most comfortable in a sitting position but seemed agitated, appeared exceedingly pale, and to be showing signs of peripheral cyanosis.

A radio call to the hospital was performed midway into the trip but was interrupted as Mr. Therion suddenly vomited. Almost at the same time he went into respiratory and cardiac arrest (cardiac monitor showing ventricular fibrillation). The driver quickly pulled off the road and went to help his partner with the patient.

He was quickly placed supine and suctioned. A CPR board was placed under his back and cardiac compression along with manual ventilation with a bag-valve mask, were given. As compression ensued so did the emesis, which continued to create airway problems. Suction was performed after each set of compressions and a number of oral airways were disposed of.

Defibrillation was indicated and delivered (200 j.) to no initial effect. A second shock (200 j.) was also unsuccessful. Finally a third shock (360 j.)

was delivered, providing an idioventricular rhythm. This rhythm, which gave a rate of about 35, was supported with continued cardiac compressions since a carotid pulse could not palpated. The patient was intubated successfully and ventilatory efforts continued. The idioventricular rhythm suddenly reverted to asystole and CPR was maintained into the ER without change in Mr. Therion's status.

Multiple-Choice Questions

1. Which of the following are considered risk factors for the development of a myocardial infarction?

1. hypertension
2. diabetes mellitus
3. chronic fatigue syndrome
4. hypercholesterolemia

   a) 1, 2, 3
   b) 1, 3, 4
   c) 2, 3, 4
   d) 1, 2, 4
   e) all of the above

2. Common medications whose presence should alert the EMT to a previous cardiac history include:

1. Dilantin
2. Digitalis
3. Diuretics
4. Diazepam

   a) 1, 2
   b) 2, 3
   c) 1, 4
   d) 2, 3, 4
   e) 1, 3, 4

3. The precipitating event in a myocardial infarction is most commonly:

a) coronary artery spasm resulting in restricted blood flow
b) acute volume overload leading to myocardial stress and failure
c) formation of a thrombus in a diseased coronary artery
d) acute respiratory failure leading to acute myocardial hypoxia
e) valvular defects resulting in micro-emboli occluding coronary arteries

4. Myocardial infarction has several complications. The most common threat(s) to life is/are:

a) dysrhythmias
b) ventricular aneurysm
c) congestive heart failure
d) cardiogenic shock
e) pericarditis

5. Starling's Law refers to an increased:

a) inotropic effect on the ventricle secondary to the release of epinephrine.
b) chronotropic effect on the ventricle secondary to the release of epinephrine.
c) contractile force of the ventricle resulting from increased thoracic pressure during CPR.
d) ventricular ejection fraction following increased diastolic filling.
e) cardiac output resulting from an increased heart rate.

6. Electrolytes play a significant role in cardiac functioning. Which of the following are true?

1. Hyponatremia decreases muscular strength.
2. Hypercalcemia increases the risk of heart block.
3. Hypocalcemia decreases myocardial contractility.
4. Hypokalemia increases myocardial irritability.

a) 1, 2, 4
b) 2, 3, 4
c) 1, 2, 3
d) 1, 3, 4
e) all of the above

7. The most common and classic symptom of a myocardial infarction is chest pain. Which of the following are true statements?

1. Substernal chest pain often radiates into the neck and/or jaw, or to the left shoulder and/or arm.
2. Pain of a myocardial infarction is often alleviated with rest, decreased anxiety, and nitroglycerin.

3. Duration of chest pain in a myocardial infarction usually exceeds thirty minutes.
4. Some elderly and/or diabetic patients when experiencing a myocardial infarction *do not* complain of chest pain.
   a) 1, 4
   b) 2, 4
   c) 1, 2, 3
   d) 1, 3, 4
   e) all of the above

8. The location of the myocardial infarct depends on the involvement of the coronary arteries. Which of the following are true?
   1. Anterior wall infarcts are usually the result of a left coronary artery occlusion.
   2. Lateral wall infarcts are usually the result of a right coronary artery occlusion.
   3. Septal wall infarcts are usually the result of a left coronary artery occlusion.
   4. Inferior wall infarcts are usually the result of a right coronary artery occlusion.
   a) 1, 4
   b) 1, 2
   c) 1, 3, 4
   d) 2, 3, 4
   e) all of the above

9. Commonly associated signs and symptoms of a myocardial infarction include:
   1. syncope
   2. ataxic respirations
   3. palpitations
   4. nausea/vomiting
   5. bradycardia
   6. tachycardia
   a) 2, 3, 4, 6
   b) 1, 3, 5, 6
   c) 1, 2, 4, 5
   d) 1, 3, 4, 5, 6
   e) all of the above

10. Which of the following statements concerning the pathophysiology of a myocardial infarction are true?

   1.   Collateral circulation may, over time, provide an overlap of blood supply to an occluded area limiting the damage caused by an MI.

   2.   Ischemia leads to necrosis, which allows connective tissue to form the remnant scar tissue.

   3.   It is the scar tissue that becomes the source and origin of many dysrhythmias.

   4.   Damaged myocardium is most vulnerable to rupture during the first one to two weeks after a myocardial infarction.

     a) 2, 3, 4
     b) 1, 2, 4
     c) 1, 3, 4
     d) 1, 2, 3
     e) all of the above

11. In differentiating a dissecting thoracic aortic aneurysm from a myocardial infarction, the patient with the former, more often:

   1.   complains of diffuse chest pain without radiation

   2.   has asymmetrical pulses

   3.   has a history of poorly controlled hypertension

   4.   will progress to the complication of cardiac tamponade

     a) 1, 2, 3
     b) 1, 3, 4
     c) 2, 3, 4
     d) 1, 2, 4
     e) all of the above

12. Initial field management of a suspected myocardial infarction includes which of the following?

   1.   Provide reassurance and ensure the patient avoids any physical exertion.

   2.   Administer oxygen 8 to 12 lpm via non-rebreather mask.

   3.   Ensure the patient remains supine in order to anticipate cardiogenic shock.

   4.   Initiate electrocardiogram (ECG) monitoring.

     a) 1, 2, 4
     b) 2, 3, 4
     c) 1, 3, 4
     d) 1, 2, 3
     e) all of the above

Debriefing

Mr. Therion's cardiovascular disease has resulted from the progressive and degenerative process known as atherosclerosis. Over a period of many years there forms a buildup of thick, hard atherosclerotic plaques referred to as atheromas, or atheromatous lesions along the arterial walls. These lesions develop as low-density lipoproteins (LDLs—the so-called bad cholesterol), adhere to the intima of the artery, and attract monocytes. The combination of the lipids becoming rancid and the response of the endothelial cells at the site allow for the formation of plaques.

With time the atheromas become fibrotic and calcified, narrowing the lumen and partially or totally obstructing the involved arteries. In many cases, collateral circulation develops over time and helps to compensate. This is one reason why many patients survive the initial insult of a complete occlusion.

The actual myocardial infarction (heart attack) most often occurs when a thrombus lodges within a coronary artery at the site of narrowing, occluding the blood flow beyond.

Whereas the mental image of a slightly obese individual with an extensive history of smoking and drinking conjured up by the ambulance crew may not be atypical, it is also possible to see a patient without many of the predisposing factors, particularly if there is a strong heritable component.

Mr. Therion's reluctance to admit that anything was seriously wrong is also not unusual. Patient denial is common. Delays in obtaining medical assistance during the first two hours (most deaths due to MIs occur in the first two hours) after the onset of signs/symptoms can be precarious. Life-threatening arrythmias most often occur during the initial stages of an MI, when myocardial ischemia produces muscular irritability and excitability.

During assessment a third heart sound (gallop) was discovered just after S2. The presence of this additional heart sound, although rare, indicates turbulent blood flowing into a less than compliant left ventricle. It occurs early in diastole and may be normal in some young people but in the presence of an MI it may be an indicator of heart failure.

With the release of adrenalin compensating for a decreasing cardiac output during a myocardial infarction we would expect the heart rate to show tachycardia, however certain arrhythmias may slow or block conduction through the A-V node and present as bradycardia. In this case there was a slight continuous delay in conduction (PR interval greater than .2 seconds) described as a first-degree heart block. ST segment elevation, which may reveal injury, would likely only be seen if the left anterior descending (LAD) coronary artery was compromised inferiorly since the cardiac monitor is usually set to lead II and only provides a look at the inferior surface of the left ventricle. Damage to the myocardium resulting from occlusion of the left coronary artery (near its take-off) including the circumflex branch and right coronary artery will not normally be seen in lead II.

Mr. Therion had taken three nitro tablets, which act to dilate coronary arteries in order to improve myocardial perfusion. In the presence of a myocardial infarction the nitroglycerin is ineffective and in this case in the presence of alcohol it may even be counterproductive. Alcohol is a peripheral vasodilator and since nitroglycerine also vasodilates peripheral blood vessels, the combination could significantly reduce venous return, decreasing cardiac output and diminishing the blood flow through the coronary sinuses. The end result is a reduction in myocardial perfusion and further ischemia, which may lead to necrosis of myocardial tissue. Most protocols for the administration of nitroglycerine ensure a systolic BP of at least 100 and a pulse of at least 60.

ASA is an analgesic, an anti-inflammatory, an antipyretic, and most important, a platelet aggregation inhibitor (reduces clotting). By preventing platelets from sticking together, ASA reduces the amount of clotting in the narrowed coronary artery of the MI victim. ASA, given in the first few hours of an acute myocardial infarction, has been shown to reduce mortality 30 percent.

Nausea and vomiting are common signs associated with an MI. After eating, the basal metabolic rate (BMR) rises slightly to accommodate digestion (increased blood flow to the abdomen), resulting in an increased heart rate and increased myocardial oxygen demands.

The tremendous anxiety associated with an MI, and the sense of impending doom that often arises, can also increase the oxygen demands and workload of the myocardium. It is therefore extremely important to make the patient as comfortable as possible, give a 100 percent concentration of oxygen, and provide reassurance throughout the call.

On a final note, without early definitive airway management through endotracheal intubation, successful resuscitation of even a witnessed arrest becomes a difficult process in the presence of an airway obstruction (copious vomiting in this case).

Follow-Up

Mr. Therion was treated as a witnessed cardiac arrest, was intubated, and received the full compliment of medications as per cardiac arrest protocol, however resuscitation was unsuccessful and he was declared dead thirty-five minutes after arrival. Autopsy results revealed an anterior wall myocardial infarction along with a ruptured ventricular aneurysm causing sudden death.

There will always be a small number of patients for whom even the best of efforts in providing emergency care and resuscitation will prove fruitless.

Fact from Fiction

An in-depth evaluation of chest pain is essential in order to differentiate between the numerous possible causes. Primary characteristics of chest pain include: factors that precipitate and relieve it; quality and severity; location and radiation; onset and duration; and associated features. Chest pain is a common symptom, which may result from a wide variety of sources, both of cardiac and non-cardiac origin.

Cardiovascular causes of chest pain include myocardial infarction, the one uppermost in minds of EMTs. MI features substernal chest pain, which may radiate to neck, jaw, shoulder, or arms (left common). Heaviness, pressure, burning, and constriction are all common descriptives for MI pain. Onset is usually acute and severe pain persists for at least thirty minutes, often longer. Pain is unrelieved by rest or nitroglycerine, and is often accompanied by shortness of breath, diaphoresis, nausea, vomiting, and weakness.

Other causes of cardiac origin include angina pectoris (reversible myocardial ischemia), which is typically brought on by exertion, and relieved by rest and nitroglycerine. Duration for angina is usually less than fifteen minutes. Unstable angina (precursor to an MI) and Prinzmetals's (Variant) angina are also forms of ischemic heart disease with a well-established history and a limited duration of chest pain. Pericarditis produces chest pain that distinguishes itself by being aggravated by movement (rotating chest) and deep breathing, and is relieved by sitting up and leaning forward. Aortic dissection, often associated with hypertension, radiates pain through to the back and is described as excruciating, knifelike, and tearing.

Chest pain of non-cardiac origin includes pulmonary embolism (PE) with pleuritic chest pain (localized over area involved) aggravated by breathing; pneumonia with pleurisy, which is similar to PE with painful breathing; spontaneous pneumothorax where chest pain is unilateral, well localized, also aggravated by breathing, and associated with hyperresonance and decreased breath sounds over involved lung; musculoskeletal disorders such as muscle pull or simple fracture of a rib, where pain is aggravated by movement and breathing, and injured area tender to pressure/palpation; esophageal reflux which is epigastric pain described as burning and aggravated by lying supine; peptic ulcer, which can be epigastric or substernal pain, is also described as burning and is relieved by antacid or bland food; gallbladder disease which is epigastric pain, usually in the right upper quadrant that often follows ingestion of fatty meals; and anxiety states whose location of chest pain often moves from place to place, and is associated with emotional stress.

Answer Key & Rationale

1. d) Hypertension, diabetes mellitus (close to 50 percent of patients with MI have a medical history that includes diabetes), and hypercholesterolemia (elevated low-density lipoproteins, or LDLs) are all considered risk factors for the development of coronary artery disease. Other risk factors include smoking, lack of exercise, excessive sodium intake, family history, advanced age, obesity, stress or a type-A personality (aggressive, overly competitive, addicted to work, chronically impatient), and previous history of heart ailment.

2. b) Digitalis (Digoxin, Lanoxin) is used for the treatment of congestive heart failure and atrial fibrillation or flutter. Diuretics (furosemide, Lasix) are used for the treatment of congestive heart failure and hypertension. Other medications that should alert the EMT include nitroglycerin and propranolol (Inderal) for the treatment of angina, as well as antihypertensives and antidysrhythmias. Many heart patients also take an aspirin daily, usually enteric ASA.

Dilantin is used to prevent seizures, and diazepam (Valium) is a minor tranquillizer.

3. c) Coronary artery spasm, circulatory overload, acute respiratory failure, and valvular effects can all precipitate an MI. However, the most common pathology involves a blood clot (thrombus) lodging or forming in a coronary artery which has been narrowed (decreased lumen diameter) through atherosclerotic plaques referred to as atheromatous lesions.

4. a) Dysrhythmias are the most common complication occurring in the few hours after the onset of symptoms. Life-threatening dysrhythmias include ventricular fibrillation (VF), ventricular tachycardia (VT), and some atrioventricular blocks. Also of note, premature ventricular complexes (PVCs) may be a forerunner to the life-threatening dysrhythmia VF.

5. d) The cardiac muscle is extensible in that it may be stretched to allow greater filling of the ventricles. Once the ventricles are filled, the tension placed on the cardiac muscle by stretching causes the myocardium to contract with greater force. The increased force of contraction is called Starling's Law. The result is an increased stroke volume, ejection fracture, and a subsequent increase in cardiac output.

6. e) In the resting state, the cell membrane is fifty to seventy-five times more permeable to potassium than to sodium ions. During depolarization the permeability to sodium increases and sodium ions rush into the cell.

As potassium leaves the cell calcium slowly enters the cell through calcium channels and triggers a release of calcium from intracellular storage sites (sarcoplasmic reticulum) initiating contraction. A calcium deficit (hypocalcemia) causes neuromuscular excitability, which will lead to weak cardiac contractions if uncorrected. Calcium excess (hypercalcemia) can lead to dysrhythmias, particularly heart block.

Too much or too little potassium causes changes in the conduction rate of nerve impulses, which can lead to dysrhythmias. Hypokalemia in particular weakens the myocardium.

7. d) The pain of an MI is most often substernal and may radiate into the neck and jaw, and/or to the left shoulder and arm (primarily the medial aspect of the left arm). Whereas anginal pain is usually alleviated within a few minutes by rest and the taking of nitroglycerin, the pain from an MI is not usually affected by anything the patient does. The pain associated with angina (coronary insufficiency) will rarely last longer than fifteen minutes; however the pain associated with an MI may persist for several hours.

Acute myocardial infarction without pain is called a "silent MI" and most often occurs among the elderly and/or diabetic patients.

Patients may also present with atypical pain, possibly shoulder, arm, neck, or jaw pain without chest pain.

8. c) The majority of myocardial infarctions involve the left ventricle which is the main pumping chamber of the heart. Coronary arteries supply blood to the heart muscle, delivering 200 to 250 ml of blood to the myocardium each minute.

The arteries are broken down into right and left with the right coronary artery supplying blood to the right atrium, right ventricle, and the inferior aspect of the left ventricle. The left main coronary artery subdivides into the left anterior descending (LAD) and the circumflex arteries. The LAD supplies the anterior wall of the left ventricle as well as the intraventricular septum. The circumflex artery feeds the lateral and posterior portions of the left ventricle, as well as part of the right ventricle.

In addition, many patients who survive an MI do so because of the many anastomoses that exist between arterioles of coronary arteries; allowing for the development of collateral circulation.

9. d) Signs and symptoms commonly seen in the presence of an MI include syncope (particularly with any decrease in cardiac output), dysrhythmias both bradycardic (predominantly inferior wall MIs with parasympathetic stimulation) and tachycardic (predominantly anterior wall MIs with sympathetic stimulation), palpitation (often with the supra ventricular tachy dysrhythmias), nausea, and vomiting.

Additional signs and symptoms other than chest pain include: severe apprehension/anxiety, agitation, confusion, diaphoresis, shortness of breath, pallor, cyanosis, a third (S3) and/or fourth (S4) heart sound, pulmonary edema, dilated pupils, fever, and fatigue.

10. b) Collateral circulation may restrict an injured area of the myocardium to ischemia and as such prevent extensive damage through necrosis.

As perfusion of cardiac cells is interrupted, the ischemia leads to anaerobic metabolism. If anaerobic metabolism is permitted to persist, the cardiac cells distal to the site of the occlusion will die (necrosis). Over the span of several weeks scar tissue comprised of connective tissue develops in the infarcted area. Scar tissue is without elasticity and cannot expand to increase diastolic filling nor has it the ability to contract, resulting in a diminished stroke volume.

It is not the infarcted necrotic area that is the source of dysrhythmias, but the area surrounding the damaged tissue. This peri-infarction area survives, but because of the ischemia, it is the origin of many dysrhythmias.

During the first couple of weeks following an extensive MI the damaged myocardium is weak and vulnerable to rupture. Decreased activity, reducing stress and excitement, are recommended during this time. The life-threatening complication would be a ruptured ventricular aneurysm.

11. c) The pain of a dissecting aortic aneurysm is most often described as sharp and tearing. Although the pain rarely radiates to the jaw and arms it often extends to the neck, shoulders, lower back, and abdomen. Pain is often more severe on the right side.

An ascending aortic aneurysm may also include unequal intensities of the right carotid and left radial pulses, as well as a difference in blood pressure between the right and left arms.

Ascending aortic aneurysm, the most common type, is seen in hypertensive men below age sixty, while the descending aortic aneurysm is seen most often in elderly hypertensive men.

An intimal tear leading back toward the heart could lead to cardiac tamponade as blood fills the pericardial sac, decreasing diastolic filling, reducing stroke volume and cardiac output.

12. a) In order to decrease myocardial oxygen demands on an already compromised myocardium it is important to: decrease anxiety through reassurance; ensure the patient does not exert himself or herself at any point; and keep the patient in a comfortable position, usually semi-sitting unless there is evidence of hemodynamic compromise.

Patients should be administered a medium to high concentration of oxygen and their ECG monitored for any life-threatening dysrhythmias.

The crew had just given their order over the outside speaker at one of their regular fast food spots when the call came in: "possible seizure at the downtown union mission." Lunch would have to wait even longer.

They extricated themselves from the line of cars and proceeded at the high priority with which the call was given out.

The new paramedic, recently recruited, commented that with any luck the seizure would be over by the time they got there and jokingly suggested that they might even slow down a little to ensure this was the case. The veteran crew member replied that he was probably right but added that it might, however, be "status."

They arrived without delay in front of an old stone building that had once served as the local jail. The conversion to soup kitchen and refuge for the homeless had taken place with minimal expense. The patient was on the second floor and there was no elevator in the building. The main stretcher was left at the foot of the stairs on the landing and a fold-out portable stretcher was taken up the two flights of stairs.

The information provided to the crew revealed that their patient, Andrew McCloud, who was still seizing, had a history of convulsions. His last seizure at the mission was about a month ago and had lasted several minutes. He had adamantly refused transport the last time and being a big man at 6'6" and 280 lbs (126 kg), few people argued with him. No further background information or related history was available.

As the medics approached they observed Mr. McCloud to be supine on a cot in a clonic stage of seizure activity. There was constant jerking of all four limbs along with an irregular pulse and noisy respirations. There were about six of his friends who were in the process of trying to hold him down. Within seconds all motion stopped and the convulsion ended.

One of those helping to restrain Mr. McCloud piped up that he "goes limp but starts up again a few minutes later." The attending paramedic determined that Mr. McCloud had been in and out of a seizure for the past twenty minutes. There was some initial delay in calling for help since his friends thought he had the DTs (delirium tremens) and was going through alcohol withdrawal and that after the initial seizure was over he would be okay.

The assessment revealed no response to painful stimuli and pupils were dilated and slow to react. Pulse was 94 regular and bounding and a blood pressure reading was 174/120. Respirations were more regular but remained noisy and rapid. He was very diaphoretic and also had urinary incontinence. Secretions were suctioned around the airway and the paramedics were in the process of providing oxygen when Mr. McCloud started seizing again.

Mr. McCloud's friends were cautioned not to continue with their restraint but to help position him on the portable stretcher strapping his trunk in as best they could. Unfortunately there was no abatement of Mr. McCloud's seizure activity during the descent down the two flights of stairs. A 280-lb. patient in full seizures being carried on an undersized cot provides a picture that needs no commentary.

The crew survived their ordeal managing to avoid the filing of workman's compensation claims on completion of the call. The patient finally stopped seizing as he was being loaded into the ambulance. He was repositioned on his left side and a more complete secondary assessment revealed no evidence of trauma, no needle tracks that might suggest drug abuse, no MedicAlert® bracelet, however a card in his wallet did indicate he suffered from post-traumatic epilepsy and that the medication Dilantin had been prescribed. One hundred percent oxygen was provided via a non-rebreather mask, an oral airway was inserted, and an IV was quickly inserted and secured.

Just as a second set of vitals was obtained, Mr. McCloud started convulsing once again. It appeared to begin with his left arm and progress rapidly to the entire body. Due to the close proximity of the hospital, the crew did not take the time to administer Ativan or Valium in the prehospital setting. The patient remained in a clonic state of seizure throughout the remainder of the call.

Multiple-Choice Questions

1. Seizures may result from:
1. hypoxia
2. hyperglycemia
3. sepsis
4. strokes

   a) 1, 2, 3
   b) 1, 2, 4
   c) 2, 3, 4
   d) 1, 3, 4
   e) all of the above

2. Seizures may result from:
   1. head trauma
   2. drug withdrawal
   3. eclampsia
   4. muscular dystrophy
      a) 1, 2, 3
      b) 1, 3, 4
      c) 1, 2, 4
      d) 2, 3, 4
      e) all of the above

3. Which of the following statements about the pathophysiology of a seizure is correct?
   a) A generalized seizure always starts in one part of the body and spreads rapidly.
   b) When a seizure occurs, neurons in the cerebral cortex rapidly communicate with other neurons by firing intermittent signals.
   c) When a seizure occurs, neurons in the cerebral cortex fire at the same time in a paroxysmal burst.
   d) The underlying neuropathophysiology of seizures is well established and most are secondary to metabolic derangement.
   e) While some seizures are idiopathic, most result from alterations in membrane permeability secondary to structural lesions.

4. Seizures are classified as partial or generalized. Partial seizures include:
   1. absence seizure
   2. myoclonic seizure
   3. temporal lobe seizure
   4. psychomotor seizure
      a) 1, 2
      b) 3, 4
      c) 1, 2, 4
      d) 2, 3, 4
      e) all of the above

5. Generalized seizures include:
   1. akinetic seizure
   2. Jacksonian seizure
   3. tonic-clonic seizure
   4. atonic seizure
      a) 1, 3
      b) 2, 3
      c) 1, 2, 4
      d) 1, 3, 4
      e) all of the above

6. Which of the following statements regarding "status epilepticus" are true?
1. It is a continuous seizure state which can occur in all seizure types.
2. It is a series of seizures without an intervening period of consciousness.
3. In the tonic-clonic form it can be life-threatening.
4. It can result from abrupt withdrawal of anti-epileptic medication.

   a) 1, 2, 3
   b) 1, 2, 4
   c) 1, 3, 4
   d) 2, 3, 4
   e) all of the above

7. Complications that often result from "status epilepticus" include:
1. hypothermia
2. cerebral hypoxia
3. hypoglycemia
4. hypotension

   a) 1, 2
   b) 2, 3
   c) 1, 2, 4
   d) 1, 3, 4
   e) all of the above

8. Signs and symptoms associated with a tonic-clonic seizure often include:
1. incontinence
2. extreme muscular rigidity
3. hypoventilation
4. diaphoresis

   a) 1, 2, 3
   b) 1, 3, 4
   c) 2, 3, 4
   d) 1, 2, 4
   e) all of the above

9. Signs and symptoms associated with a tonic-clonic seizure often include:
1. warning sensation
2. cyanosis
3. tachycardia
4. salivation

   a) 1, 2, 3
   b) 1, 2, 4
   c) 2, 3, 4
   d) 1, 3, 4
   e) all of the above

10. Signs and symptoms associated with the "postictal" phase of a seizure include:
    1. severe headache
    2. confusion, disorientation
    3. transient hemiparesis
    4. severe fatigue
        a) 1, 2, 4
        b) 2, 3, 4
        c) 1, 3, 4
        d) 1, 2, 3
        e) all of the above

11. Seizure management should include:
    1. patient restraint to avoid self-inflicted injury
    2. always ensuring the insertion of a bite block to prevent the patient from biting his or her tongue
    3. placement in the lateral recumbent position
    4. withholding supplemental oxygen, since seizure patients have been hyperventilating and are at risk for carpal-pedal spasms
        a) 3
        b) 1, 2
        c) 1, 4
        d) 2, 3, 4
        e) 1, 3, 4

12. Seizure management should also include:
    1. allowing the convulsion to be witnessed by a number of people so that the description may be corroborated
    2. ensuring the patient faces the fact that they are an epileptic since they have no memory of the event
    3. having only one person communicating with the patient during the postictal phase
    4. never allowing the patient to sleep following a seizure since they may fall into a coma
        a) 3
        b) 1, 2
        c) 1, 2, 4
        d) 2, 3, 4
        e) 1, 3, 4

Debriefing

Most seizures are over by the time prehospital providers arrive at the scene and for this reason it is important that a detailed description of the seizure activity be compiled. Relevant information includes whether the patient expressed any prodromal symptoms prior to the seizure, such as unusual smells, queasiness, or auditory or visual cues that a seizure might be imminent. This is a subjective sensation known as an aura, which is often the same repeating signature for the patient prior to each seizure.

In a tonic-clonic seizure (formally called a grand mal seizure), loss of consciousness quickly follows the aura and it is important to determine from witnesses whether there was any accidental head trauma during this phase. With a little warning, usually the patient will lie down.

Extreme rigidity characterizes the tonic phase and the eyes of the patient may deviate away from the site of the irritating lesion. If the seizure is a simple partial and subsequently spreads to a generalized seizure it is important to find out which part of the body was affected first as this may indicate the site of irritation.

The clonic phase represents the actual convulsion represented by alterations in muscular rigidity and relaxation or, as is often described, uncontrolled jerking of limbs and body.

Management of seizures includes protecting the patient by clearing the area, helping to keep the patient from accidentally hitting nearby objects. The patient should not be restrained, first because no matter what is done the patient is going to convulse, and second because any restraining actions could seriously injure muscles, bones, or joints.

It is helpful to find out how long the convulsion lasted, since the complications resulting from seizures are compounded by time. Most tonic-clonic seizures usually have a duration of between two and five minutes. Remember that during times of extreme stress, such as waiting for an ambulance, time itself may be distorted for witnesses, to whom each minute may seem like five.

Despite the fact that most seizures are over before EMS arrives and often occur among known epileptics, the seizure may be only the secondary problem. The primary event could be extremely serious, particularly if it is the result of eclampsia, barbiturate withdrawal, recent head trauma, hypoglycemia, carbon monoxide poisoning, meningitis, or encephalitis. In addition, any seizure occurring for the first time or seizures occurring among children should receive a high priority and be fully investigated.

In summary, for seizures that are over before EMS arrives, gaining a complete and detailed description of the event can be one of the most important factors in the management of the call. Simple details such as the side to which the eyes deviate (usually away from the irritating focus) can help locate the problem's origin.

Many patients who suffer from epilepsy often refuse transport but should nonetheless be encouraged to seek medical attention emphasizing the importance of having antiepileptic drug blood levels checked at regular intervals. Remember also that patients during the postictal phase (recovery stage of tonic-clonic) of the seizure are tired, confused, and sometimes unintentionally uncooperative or combative. The paramedics should remain with the patient until he or she is fully oriented and capable of making sound decisions.

Status epilepticus on the other hand is a true emergency and will lead to hypoglycemia, hypoxia, acidosis, and ultimately brain damage if there is no intervention. If definitive care is not to be immediately provided at scene, rapid transport of the "status" patient becomes the priority.

Aside from recognition of the need for rapid transport, an important intervention goal is always to protect the patient from airway obstruction and to deliver 100 percent oxygen. During a prolonged seizure air exchange is generally ineffective since the normal ventilatory mechanisms of the patient are seriously impaired. Once the airway has been maintained, ventilatory assistance can be accomplished through a bag-valve mask providing increased oxygenation during periods of hypopnea and apnea.

The most common cause of status epilepticus remains failure to take prescribed anticonvulsant medication, although other precipitating factors should not be ruled out.

Follow-Up

Once in the hospital, the patient was diagnosed to be in "status epilepticus" and was given stat IV doses of phenytoin and diazepam to little effect, which necessitated the introduction of IV barbiturates. The seizures finally did stop, however Mr. McCloud remained unresponsive and was intubated. Blood glucose levels indicated hypoglycemia. He was given a 100 mg thiamine (slow intravenous infusion) along with 50 percent dextrose bolus followed by D5W. Oxygen was administered in high concentrations and ventilation supported with a bag-valve device.

Mr. McCloud regained consciousness and was eventually released from the hospital. It was discovered he had been in a car accident years earlier and suffered traumatic head injury, which left him prone to seizures. They had initially been fairly well controlled but social factors—the loss of his job, abuse of alcohol, and deteriorating home life— were affecting his compliance with medication. Alcohol abuse was also leading to an increasing frequency of seizure activity.

Fact from Fiction

Epilepsy ranks second among the most common neurological disorders, surpassed only by strokes. Epilepsy is either "primary," where no structural or metabolic abnormality can be found (also termed idiopathic), or it is "secondary," with an established etiology. In all cases, whether there is a brain tumor, lesion, structural malformation, electrolyte imbalance, drug overdose, drug withdrawal, meningitis, eclampsia, cerebral hypoxia, or head injury, the seizure activity is due to an abnormal alteration in certain neurons, which create both hyperactivity and hypersensitivity.

In generalized tonic-clonic seizures, a sudden explosion of high-voltage, high frequency activity can be seen over the entire cortex on an EEG. The rapid-fire discharge of neuronal activity usually has a starting point (epileptogenic focus), which recruits adjacent neurons and spreads over both hemispheres.

Several hours before an attack, a prodromal warning may take place. A mood change, insomnia, loss of appetite, upset stomach, palpitations, or just a sense of apprehension may provide some warning of an impending seizure.

An indication that a seizure is just about to take place is called an aura. The aura, which occurs in about half of all cases, is usually sensory and is distinct for each individual. If an aura is experienced at the start of a seizure, it can be a useful clue to the location of the epitogenic focus. The Canadian neurosurgeon Dr. Wilder Penfield led the way in mapping the brain when treating epileptics by localizing the irritating focus through the use of tiny electrical stimulation to areas of the brain, while the patient remained conscious.

Once the paroxysms of neuronal discharge move outward from the localized area and spread to the thalamus and reticular activating system (RAS), loss of consciousness results. In the initial phase of the seizure the body goes rigid (tonic), with jaw snapping shut (tongue may be bitten), and as the diaphragm and chest muscles are seized in spasm, air is forced out through closed vocal cords emitting a high pitched cry. At this point the individual is apneic and turning cyanotic. Bowel and/or bladder control may be lost at this stage.

The next phase is the rapid jerking of limbs, where rhythmic and rather violent muscular contractions are taking place. Frothy saliva appears at the mouth, sweating is profuse, and stertorous breathing completes the picture. After a few minutes, the convulsion subsides and the noisy ineffective breathing gives way to a deep inspiratory sigh (the result of an accumulation of carbon dioxide).

During the final phase (postictal), as the individual comes to, he or she is limp, exhausted, totally confused, and often wants to be left alone to sleep for several hours. A subsequent headache and understandably sore muscles may be the only residual aftereffects of the experience.

Although some individuals are prone to seizures given a lower-than-normal threshold, they can occur in anyone, given the right conditions.

Answer Key & Rationale

1. d); **2.** a)   Seizures can have a wide variety of causes, including anoxia and cerebral hypoxia from any cause; sepsis particularly when combined with pyrexia; strokes (cerebrovascular accidents); head trauma recent or past; drug withdrawal including alcohol; eclampsia (toxemia of pregnancy); brain tumors; meningitis and encephalitis; hypoglycemia; ingestion of toxins (mercury, lead, or carbon monoxide); as well as idiopathic origin.

3. c)   Normally, neurons in the brain's cerebral cortex communicate with each other by firing electrochemical signals. The firing is limited to certain areas and groups of neurons depending on the activity and tasks needed to be performed. During a seizure the neurons fire simultaneously in one paroxysmal burst. There is no communication between neurons since they are all trying to get their information across without anyone listening.

A partial seizure may start in one part of the body and spread to become a generalized seizure.

Since the underlying cause of most seizures remains idiopathic, the neuropathophysiology is not well understood.

4. b) Partial seizures occur in 80 percent of people who have seizures. A partial seizure is local in origin and always starts in only one part of the cerebral cortex, although it may spread to become a generalized seizure.

A temporal lobe seizure or simple partial seizure is often confined to an uncontrollable shaking in a foot or hand, or it may be that the mouth twitches. It usually lasts no more than a minute. A psychomotor seizure or complex partial seizure also has focal disturbances, such as repetitive fidgeting with cloths, lip smacking, aimless wandering, or unexplained rage. There is some impairment of consciousness as well.

Absence (petit mal) seizure is a generalized seizure usually lasting less than fifteen seconds and consisting of a blank stare. Myoclonic is also a generalized seizure with uncontrolled motor movement, a generalized jerking of an extremity usually lasting only a few seconds.

5. d) A tonic-clonic seizure, formerly called a grand mal seizure, involves the entire cerebral cortex. The patient remains unconscious throughout the seizure and because the entire brain is affected, he or she won't feel or see anything during the seizure or remember anything afterward.

During an atonic seizure, sometimes called an akinetic seizure, the patient experiences a loss of consciousness and a loss of muscle tone, usually resulting in a fall.

A Jacksonian seizure is a focal motor seizure known as a simple partial seizure.

6. e) Status seizures are those that do not abate on their own and require medical intervention. Status epilepticus most often results from abrupt withdrawal of antiepileptic medication. The seizures may be continuous or a
series of seizures occurring without an intervening period of consciousness. Tonic-clonic status seizures can be fatal if drug intervention is not
provided immediately.

7. b) Status epilepticus is a medical emergency that requires prompt aggressive treatment. Any delay can lead to cerebral hypoxia combined with
an increased oxygen consumption and inadequate ventilation; additionally, hypoglycemia results as glucose is rapidly depleted from the
vascular system. Status patients are also at risk of developing hyperthermia, hypertension, increased intracranial pressure, fractures of the
long bones and of the spine, severe dehydration, and necrosis of the
cardiac muscles.

8. d); **9.** e)   Signs and symptoms commonly associated with tonic-clonic
seizures include incontinence (urinary and/or bowel), extreme rigidity
(tonic) of muscles, diaphoresis, warning sensation (aura), cyanosis, tachycardia, and salivation. Also included may be an epileptic cry, labored
breathing, apnea, and tongue-biting.

10. e) Once consciousness is regained following a tonic-clonic seizure, confusion, disorientation, extreme fatigue, and a severe headache are common
symptoms. Although less common, a transient hemiparesis (Todd's
paralysis) may also be present. These symptoms will abate over a time
period which may last from minutes to hours.

11. a); **12.** a)   In the management of a seizure, the patient should be positioned
on his or her side if possible to prevent aspiration. There should never be
any attempt at restraining the patient (unless the patient is in status
epilepticus and a minimal amount of restraint is required for transport)
since there is really no need to restrain and doing so may injure muscles,
bones and joints. Once a seizure has commenced any possible damage to
the tongue by biting is likely to have already taken place. There is also a
risk that the patient may damage teeth if a solid object is inserted into the
mouth or that the object may be bitten through and aspirated.

Oxygen is always beneficial to anyone who is at risk for hypoxia.
During a seizure the extreme energy output from muscular activity creates
a situation where oxygen is consumed at a rate of 60 percent above the
norm. High concentrations of oxygen may be of little value for seizures of
short duration; however the use of oxygen is not contraindicated. If the
EMTs are witness to a seizure there is no need for a group of spectators.
Provide privacy by clearing the room or the area.

Because of the confusion and disorientation that occurs during the
postictal phase, there should be only one person talking to the patient.
One person speaking in a calm and reassuring voice will decrease the sen-

sory overload and lessen the chance the patient may be uncooperative or even combative.

Patients are extremely exhausted following a seizure and may just want to sleep. The patient when transported to the hospital may be allowed to sleep without fear that he or she will fall into a coma.

CASE STUDY 17

The ambulance crew was cruising slowly down Elgin Street. The call came during what was becoming a protracted debate on the finer points of gourmet coffee and which of the local establishments on Elgin Street would be their next stop. Loyalty to their favorite brand of coffee was an issue that no one took lightly.

The call however, brought them back to reality: "a six-year-old in severe respiratory distress." The information and times were recorded, lights and sirens turned on. and their favorite haunts along Elgin Street quickly receded behind them. Within five minutes they arrived at their destination, pulling up in front of a row of townhouses. The crew was met by a young girl, ten-year-old Alex, who directed them to the kitchen. The mother, Mrs. Moore, was supporting an obviously sick looking child, Timmy, who was seated on the kitchen table. A third child, three-year-old Evelyn, sat close by looking very sleepy.

It was just after 10:00 P.M. and the children had been in bed for an hour when Timmy started crying and complaining of a sore throat. Mrs. Moore thought he might be getting a slight chest cold earlier but when he had gone to bed he was without complaints. She brought Timmy to the kitchen and was giving him some hot chocolate when he complained of pain on swallowing and he started having difficulty breathing. Mrs. Moore's husband was working shift work, and since Timmy seemed to be getting visibly worse she decided to call 911.

The medics noticed that Timmy was perched on the edge of the table leaning forward, mouth open but no longer crying, all efforts seemingly concentrated on breathing. His color was pale, he had his hands on knees leaning forward with neck hyperextended, and he emitted a high-pitched sound with each inspiration.

The attending paramedic spoke to Timmy at eye level, in a calm reassuring voice, explaining who he was, and that they had some oxygen for him, which would help him breath easier. Twelve liters per minute by non-rebreather mask was given but Timmy became anxious when the mask was attached so his mom was allowed to hold it close to his face without actual contact. Timmy was connected to the cardiac monitor, which showed sinus tachycardia at a rate of 120, his respirations were 30, blood pressure was 100/64, and he was hot and diaphoretic. A pulse oximeter was clipped to Timmy's finger and indicated an O^2 sat. of 93 percent.

On auscultation the lungs sounded clear without wheezes, and other than an episode of bronchiolitis as an infant, Timmy had no previous history of asthma.

The attending paramedic briefly conferred with his partner, stating he suspected epiglottitis and that the partial airway obstruction that now existed could close off at anytime. The decision was made to transport without delay, bringing mother, who was a calming influence on Timmy, and the two other children as well.

En route, Timmy was allowed to maintain his position of comfort: seated, leaning forward, neck extended. But his breathing, despite being given humidified oxygen, did not seem to be improving. His color was turning from pale to ashen, his O^2 sat. had dropped to 87 percent, and his pulse had increased to 140. Along with decreasing breath sounds on auscultation all signs were pointing to increasing airway obstruction. Fortunately, the hospital was close.

A radio call quickly apprised the emergency room staff of the Children's Hospital of the seriousness of their young patient's condition and within minutes, without further change in status, they pulled up in front of the ER.

Multiple-Choice Questions

1. Which of the following statements concerning epiglottitis are true?
    1. The disease is usually associated with Haemophilus influenzae type B.
    2. Streptococcus, pneumococcus, and staphylococcus organisms have been implicated.
    3. Edema and swelling of the epiglottis are caused by an acute viral infection.
    4. The disease is commonly associated with parainfluenza virus types 1 and 2.

       a) 1, 2
       b) 2, 3
       c) 1, 3
       d) 2, 4
       e) 3, 4

2. The ages most commonly associated with epiglottitis are:
   a) 1 to 3
   b) 2 to 5
   c) 3 to 7
   d) 4 to 9
   e) 5 to 11

3. In differentiating epiglottitis from croup (laryngotracheobronchitis), the latter commonly:
   1. occurs in children between the ages of six months and three years
   2. occurs during the late fall and winter months
   3. is associated with a history of upper respiratory tract infection
   4. is associated with hoarseness and a "barking seal" like cough

    a) 1, 2, 3
    b) 1, 3, 4
    c) 1, 2, 4
    d) 2, 3, 4
    e) all of the above

4. Distinguishing clinical features in the presentation of epiglottitis include:
   1. excessive salivation
   2. low grade fever
   3. slow onset
   4. dysphagia

    a) 1, 2
    b) 2, 4
    c) 1, 4
    d) 3, 2
    e) 1, 3

5. Signs and symptoms seen in epiglottitis include:
   1. asymptomatic prior to onset
   2. muffled voice
   3. sitting upright leaning forward
   4. mouth open, tongue protruding

    a) 1, 2, 3
    b) 1, 2, 4
    c) 2, 3, 4
    d) 1, 3, 4
    e) all of the above

6. Signs and symptoms of epiglottitis also include:

1. stridor
2. irritability
3. flared nostrils
4. inspiratory retractions

   a) 1, 2, 4
   b) 1, 3, 4
   c) 1, 2, 3
   d) 2, 3, 4
   e) all of the above

7. In terms of growth and development, children in the age bracket who are most susceptible to epiglottitis:

1. will readily talk to strangers
2. have vivid imaginations
3. rarely have temper tantrums
4. may view treatment procedures as hostile

   a) 1, 2
   b) 2, 4
   c) 3, 4
   d) 1, 2, 3
   e) 1, 3, 4

8. When dealing with children of the age in question:

1. It is all right to lie to protect them.
2. They are often immodest at this age.
3. The child should never be told what is wrong.
4. You must rely on the parents to fill in gaps in information.

   a) 4
   b) 1, 2
   c) 2, 4
   d) 1, 2, 3
   e) 1, 3, 4

9. Within the age bracket commonly associated with epiglottitis, common illnesses and accidents include:
1. child abuse
2. asthma
3. poisonings
4. bronchiolitis
5. ingestion of foreign bodies
6. meningitis
   a) 1, 3, 4, 5
   b) 2, 3, 5, 6
   c) 1, 2, 4, 6
   d) 1, 2, 3, 5, 6
   e) all of the above

10. Occlusion of the airway can occur suddenly in epiglottitis and may be precipitated by:
1. minor irritation of the throat
2. aggravation and anxiety
3. lying the patient down
4. ingestion of a hot beverage
   a) 1, 2, 4
   b) 1, 2, 3
   c) 1, 3, 4
   d) 2, 3, 4
   e) all of the above

11. In assessing the child with suspected epiglottitis it is important to:
1. provide supplemental oxygen
2. inspect the throat to confirm an edematous bright red epiglottis
3. provide reassurance and decrease anxiety
4. consider transporting stat
   a) 1, 2, 3
   b) 1, 2, 4
   c) 2, 3, 4
   d) 1, 3, 4
   e) all of the above

12. Management of the child with epiglottitis should include:

    1. placing the child supine in order to anticipate manual ventilation
    2. administering humidified oxygen
    3. informing the receiving hospital of patient status
    4. provision of high-pressure manual ventilation if total obstruction occurs by depressing the pop-off valve on the bag-valve-mask device

        a) 1, 3, 4
        b) 2, 3, 4
        c) 1, 2, 4
        d) 1, 2, 3
        e) all of the above

Debriefing

Epiglottitis is an acute inflammation of the epiglottis, which can quickly lead to total airway obstruction. Early recognition is critical since epiglottitis can prove fatal if treatment is delayed.

Epiglottitis usually results from an infection with the bacteria Haemophilus influenzae type B. Although the primary site of infection is the epiglottis, the inflammation may spread above and below to involve the trachea and bronchi. In this situation the inflammatory edema increases the respiratory distress leading to a life-threatening airway obstruction.

Acute epiglottitis, as the name suggests, comes on suddenly with little or no warning. The child often goes to bed asymptomatic and wakens a short while after complaining of a sore throat and dysphagia. The child is often febrile and is typically found sitting upright leaning forward with neck hyperextended (tripod position). This 'turtle neck' posturing facilitates respirations. Subsequently drooling (excessive salivation), which is secondary to the dysphagia, may be seen and is an ominous sign of impending airway obstruction.

Audible inspiratory stridor (high-pitched crowing noises as air rushes through a narrowed lumen) may be present with epiglottitis along with sternal retractions and nasal flaring. The child appears apprehensive, agitated, pale, and as the obstruction worsens, the signs of hypoxemia and hypoxia including cyanosis become more pronounced.

Never attempt to visualize the airway or lay the patient supine since it may trigger laryngospasm and cause respiratory collapse. Care should also be taken not to roughly manipulate the neck area containing the swollen epiglottis since it may cause an immediate vasovagal response and cardiorespiratory arrest.

The emergency room should be notified in all instances of rapidly increasing obstruction. If the EMTs are not paramedics with the skill of intubation, the hospital staff must be prepared to provide definitive airway management. Even under the best of circumstances intubation, if required, will be difficult due to the swelling and a tracheotomy may need to be performed. Complete airway obstruction can occur within two to five hours after onset.

During transport the child should remain in the Fowler position (sitting upright) and humidified oxygen at high concentration provided. If the child is too anxious and panicky about the restriction of a facial mask, then don't force the issue. Increasing the child's anxiety level will serve only to aggravate the problem. If a complete airway obstruction and respiratory arrest does occur before intubation can be secured, then manual ventilation should be initiated. It may seem futile with a complete obstruction, however some oxygen may still get through if enough pressure is used, which may be possible if the pressure release valve for the child BVM (bag-valve-mask) is blocked off.

Epiglottitis is a true life-threatening emergency and transportation to the ER should be conducted without delay, however whenever possible try and include the other family members in the care provided. Reassuring the parents as well as other family members may have the collateral effect of decreasing the anxiety level of the patient.

Follow-Up

The emergency room staff, along with several residents, including anesthesiology, were on hand for Timmy's arrival. Lateral neck x-rays revealed a classic "thumbprint sign" (swollen epiglottis that looks like a thumbprint) confirming acute epiglottitis. A throat examination, which may well have confirmed a large, edematous, bright red epiglottis, was not performed for fear of completely occluding the airway. Timmy did not show significant improvement and intubation was required.

Throat cultures revealed an upper respiratory tract infection caused by the bacterium Haemophillus influenzae type B. Timmy received fluids for dehydration and a ten-day course of parenteral antibiotic therapy with cephalosporin.

Timmy was transferred to the pediatric intensive care unit where a decrease in the swelling of his epiglottis was finally seen late in the second day. He remained intubated, however, until his epiglottis returned to normal size. Timmy was later released without further sequelae.

Fact from Fiction

Upper respiratory infections (URI) are the most common of all diseases. They are even more common in children, with the majority in North America having at least six URIs a year. The frequency can be related to many factors, including lack of acquired immunity, increased incidence among children in day-care centers, and an increased incidence among children whose parents smoke (the predisposing factor is a deficiency of antibody-immunoglobin A, induced by cigarette smoke).

Most URIs are due to viral infections and are for the most part self-limiting, with symptoms subsiding in ten days to two weeks even without treatment. Remember, antibiotics are not helpful in the treatment of viral infection and overuse can lead to an increase in drug resistant strains of bacteria.

Epiglottitis can be viral, but it is primarily caused by the bacterial agent Haemophilus influenzae type B (Hib). The Hib vaccine has been significant in reducing the number of cases seen in children.

URI is rarely fatal, however in the case of epiglottitis the epiglottis is shaped differently in children so that even a small amount of swelling can produce respiratory distress. The diameter of the airway in a child is not only smaller, but the mucous membrane is much more vascular. Edema and swelling can totally close the airway within six to twelve hours, making epiglottitis a life-threatening emergency.

The infecting agent settles in the supraglottic area, causing rapid and potentially fatal inflammation with swelling. In cases where inflammation spreads below the epiglottis to involve the trachea and bronchi, respiratory distress is more severe and the prognosis less favorable.

The child often presents in a "sniffing dog" position. Leaning forward helps keep the airway patent and the child will usually resist any attempt to be placed in a supine position. The risk of laryngeal spasm is also minimized in the forward position. With an inability to swallow, drooling becomes a classic sign to look for. In smaller children whose accessory muscles are not well developed, "head bobbing" indicates a desperate attempt to gulp air. Every effort and all energy is concentrated on breathing, such that one look at a child with respiratory distress due to epiglottitis will stimulate the need to act promptly. A child with epiglottitis "looks sick"!

Answer Key & Rationale

1. a) The organism causing epiglottitis is most often found to be the bacteria Haemophilus influenzae type B. Occasionally pneumococci staphylococcus and group A streptococci have also been known to cause epiglottitis.

Because Haemophilus influenzae type B may cause other serious illnesses, the child may need vaccination (or revaccination) against H. influenzae.

The parainfluenza virus is often implicated in the cause of croup.

2. c) Epiglottitis can strike at any age; even into adulthood, however it most often affects children between the ages of three and seven.

Croup, which is most often caused by a viral infection, affects a slightly younger age group than epiglottitis.

3. e) Acute laryngotracheobronchitis is the most common form of croup and is usually caused by a viral infection. It commonly occurs in young children during the winter months. There is often a history of an upper respiratory tract infection and croup often flares up at night. The child typically awakens with a characteristic barking brassy cough.

It should be noted that croup is a collection of diseases under which epiglottitis is sometimes classified, along with viral croup, acute laryngitis, and laryngotracheobronchitis (LTB).

4. c) Often one of the first symptoms with which epiglottitis presents is a sore throat with dysphagia (painful swallowing). One ominous sign of increasing inflammation and edema is copious drooling, the result of pooled saliva secondary to dysphagia.

The onset of epiglottitis is most often acute with the child commonly going to bed asymptomatic. Whereas most forms of croup are associated with a low-grade fever, epiglottitis presents with a sudden high fever.

5. e); **6.** e) As mentioned above, the child may be asymptomatic prior to onset, and although often extremely anxious is not usually crying. All efforts are going into breathing as is evidenced through flared nostrils and inspiratory retractions of intercostal muscles. If able to speak the voice is muffled and the child is usually found in a turtle-neck or tripod position. This means the child is seated leaning forward with the neck hyperextended forward, mouth open, and tongue protruding.

In addition the child may be gasping or gulping for air, extremely frightened, tachypnic, and cyanotic. This is a patient who looks extremely ill.

7. b) Between the ages of three and five there is rapid development of fine and gross motor skills. Language is also showing great improvement; however the child who may know how to talk often may be too shy to say a word. The child has a vivid imagination and may be afraid. At this age they may not be receptive to treatment and will usually have a temper.

8. a) The best approach when dealing with children is to be honest and explain simply what you are doing and what is going to be done. Because of the tremendous empathy that paramedics experience when dealing with children, maintaining an objective focus in the face of life-threatening illness or injury becomes all the more challenging. Children are often anxious and fearful. As with all patients, however, it is important to establish a rapport and gain their trust.

Inaccuracies in information may be due to the child's time frame being off. Help in gathering information can be elicited from the parents. It is

(partial left page)

Questions

domen includes:

...

re true regarding penetrating trauma?
e, muscle, and liver sustain more
uch as lungs.
nce a bullet enters the body, its trajec-
e.
the abdomen should be

e chest or back while wearing a flak
um risk for injury.

e peritoneal space and the
g are located in the peritoneal

(right page)

important to listen well to the parents since they know their children better than anyone.

Allow the child to sit on the parent's lap if possible (non-life-threatening situations) when gathering information since the child will feel more protected and despite being shy may be more willing to divulge information.

If possible transport the parent with the patient.

9. d) Children within the ages that are commonly seen with epiglottitis, that is ages three to seven, are also susceptible to child abuse, asthma, poisonings, ingestion or aspiration of foreign objects, and meningitis to name just a few.

Bronchiolitis, a viral infection that mimics asthma, is most often seen in children under two years of age.

10. e) Total airway obstruction occurs in about 10 percent of cases with epiglottitis and may be brought on if the patient is made to lie down, if there is undue anxiety created, and also if there is an aggressive manual evaluation of the throat and neck. Increased inflammation and edema occluding the airway may also occur with the ingestion of a hot liquid such as hot chocolate.

11. d); **12.** b) The child may present with his or her mouth open, however no attempt should ever be made to visualize the airway since severe laryngospasm and increased swelling may result, leading to complete obstruction and respiratory arrest.

Placing the child supine while he or she is breathing may result in further occlusion of the airway. The child should be kept in the preferred position of comfort, which usually means sitting up leaning forward neck extended.

Oxygen should be provided, however the restrictive nature of a nonrebreathing mask may increase the patient's anxiety level. If the patient will not tolerate the mask it should not be forced on him or her.

The receiving hospital should always be alerted in order to prepare for intubation (if not already performed in the field) and possible tracheotomy.

Reassurance should be provided to patient and family members, and transportation to hospital should be stat.

Finally, in the management of small children many emergency services have a teddy bear program where a stuffed animal is provided to frightened children in order to minimize the traumatic experience of being taken to the hospital by ambulance.

CASE STUDY 18

911 RESPONSE: multiple shooting, victims unknown

As a veteran paramedic she was tired, not because it was late afternoon, nor because of the steady stream of calls—she was tired of listening to her partner defend and make excuses for Branden once again. Branden worked on D platoon, which was opposite their shift, which meant that her partner rarely got to see Branden. She thought this was just as well, since her partner's off-and-on relationship with Branden was nothing short of volatile.

To the veteran medic, Branden was a classic case of burn-out. She made it a point to stay upbeat and positive, despite the tough times management seemed to be giving everyone these days. Their contract was up for renewal and it looked like some benefits were going to be cut with very little forthcoming in the way of a pay raise. Just cause or not she couldn't stand the way Branden was so negative about everything. She tried to ignore him, but there was no escaping the inevitable gauntlet of negative commentary toward management, the job, and life in general, both at the beginning when they were coming on shift and he was finishing, and at the end when they were getting off and he was starting. What really concerned her was that she felt sure his attitude was spilling over into his patient care.

The veteran was just about to tell her partner to give it a rest, when call from dispatch broke through: "Possible shooting, victims unknown

Police were already on the scene, a major high tech company wi several hundred employees. Access to the building was controlled police, who allowed the ambulance to drive to a secured area. The were provided with special protective vests and informed the tac squad was already in the building. They had recently completed training exercise with the police tactical squad and they knew tight and wait. While waiting for the situation to resolve they stretcher and ensured their IV equipment and trauma kit we stocked and ready for quick access. As they were preparing ambulances and a supervisor arrived. Word was circulating well be multiple casualties. Employees under the control were now spilling out of the main entrance and two add Crackling through the portable handheld radio came th the police for the medics to be escorted in.

A sense of urgency enveloped the crews as they were taken to the fourth floor lobby. There, they were witness to seven victims including the

Multiple-Choice

assa
on
th
v

1. Rapid trauma survey of the abd
  1. assess tenderness
  2. auscultate bowel sounds
  3. assess rigidity
  4. assess distention
  a) 1, 3
  b) 2, 4
  c) 2, 3, 4
  d) 1, 3, 4
  e) all of the above

2. Which of the following statements a
  1. Highly dense organs such as bon damage than less-dense organs s
  2. A key factor to remember is that o tory will always be in a straight lir
  3. Patients with missile penetration t transported stat.
  4. Personnel who have been shot in th jacket (bulletproof vest) are at minin
  a) 1, 3
  b) 1, 2
  c) 2, 3, 4
  d) 1, 3, 4
  e) 1, 2, 3

3. The abdomen is divided into two spaces, th retroperitoneal space. Which of the followin space?
  1. pancreas
  2. liver
  3. spleen
  4. stomach
  a) 1, 2, 3
  b) 1, 3, 4
  c) 1, 2, 4
  d) 2, 3, 4
  e) all of the above

4. Which of the following are located in the retroperitoneal space?
1. bladder
2. gallbladder
3. kidneys
4. abdominal aorta

   a) 1, 2, 4
   b) 2, 3, 4
   c) 1, 3, 4
   d) 1, 2, 3
   e) all of the above

5. Assessment of the abdomen should be completed keeping in mind which of the following statements?
1. Signs of intra-abdominal injury usually appear quickly.
2. Abdominal tenderness is an unreliable indicator of injury in a patient with altered level of consciousness.
3. Auscultation and percussion are keys to abdominal assessment.
4. Using a gloved hand, it is important to probe the entry wound in an attempt to extract the bullet if no exit wound can be found.

   a) 2
   b) 1, 3
   c) 1, 2, 4
   d) 1, 3, 4
   e) 2, 3, 4

6. Signs of decompensating shock can reasonably be expected to be occurring for an otherwise healthy adult, when the systolic blood pressure drops below:

   a) 120 mmHg
   b) 110 mmHg
   c) 100 mmHg
   d) 90 mmHg
   e) 80 mmHg

7. Abdominal injuries that often go undetected include trauma to the:
1. stomach
2. pancreas
3. small intestine
4. colon

   a) 2
   b) 1, 2
   c) 2, 3, 4
   d) 1, 3, 4
   e) all of the above

8. Areas affected in abdominal injuries sustained as a result of rib fractures include:
1. diaphragm
2. liver
3. spleen
4. stomach

    a) 1
    b) 1, 2
    c) 2, 3
    d) 1, 2, 3
    e) all of the above

9. A bullet passing through a hollow organ in the abdomen, bringing about a leakage or spillage of its contents into the peritoneal cavity, can result in which of the following complications?
1. sepsis
2. peritonitis
3. septic shock
4. massive infection

    a) 4
    b) 1, 2
    c) 2, 3
    d) 1, 3, 4
    e) all of the above

10. The most reliable indicator of intra-abdominal bleeding in the absence of an obvious source is:
    a) rebound tenderness
    b) abdominal distention
    c) guarding and rigidity
    d) signs of shock
    e) external bruising

11. The classification of hemorrhagic shock is specified according to the magnitude of blood loss. There are four classes, where Class I is less than _____ percent blood loss and Class IV is greater than _____ percent blood loss.
    a) 5–30
    b) 10–35
    c) 15–40
    d) 20–45
    e) 30–50

Management of hemorrhagic shock is aimed at controlling bleeding and restoring fluid volume. The most appropriate solutions delivered in the field are:

1. D_5W
2. .9 NaCl
3. Ringer's lactate
4. plasma

    a) 1, 2
    b) 2, 3
    c) 1, 4
    d) 2, 4
    e) 1, 3

Debriefing

When shootings occur and security of the scene is at issue, for the EMS provider there is a lot of hurry up and wait. All emergency services, police, fire, and ambulance have specific roles to perform; however in order to coordinate their activities and work as a team, they have to have a basic understanding of each other's jobs. Today, as a greater number of emergency services are amalgamating there exists an excellent opportunity for cross-training. Understanding each other's roles allows for mutual respect and an appreciation of the difficulties each service faces. What results is a smooth operation, minimizing major security liability issues, and the minor issues of stepping on toes or egos.

Cooperation amongst emergency services is also extended to the aftermath of a call, where critical incident stress debriefing (CISD) sessions are conducted together with personnel involved in the incident from all services. Not only is post-traumatic stress relief addressed, but the opportunity to bond as a group generates a positive sense of teamwork.

Once they are permitted to enter the scene, the paramedics have to be prepared to react quickly. Gloves should be on and safety glasses within easy reach (blood splashes to the eyes, although rare, are a justified precaution since uncontrolled bleeding is likely when a shooting has occurred).

On entry, despite well-founded confidence in the police tactical squad to secure the scene, it is still important to do a quick assessment for hazards. Experience teaches that no two situations are identical and the only common thread is unpredictability. Once the scene is secure, when multiple victims are involved it becomes a triage situation, with the first step being confirmation the number of patients and ensuring that whatever resources in equipment personnel are identified and requested. Usually this falls to the superviso scene, but it may also be role of the first EMT to arrive.

Mass casualties or not, the case still requires the same profes approach to assessment and care. Identify yourself to your patient an your purpose. The trust and respect you gain on first impressions wasted, and allows a platform from which you can maintain patient co

Next, an initial trauma survey, conducted within a couple of minutes at most, should enable the EMT to determine the need for "load-and-go."

"Load-and-go" does not mean that you simply throw your patient on the gurney and take off. Critical management interventions are completed on scene and include ensuring and maintaining airway and ventilation; controlling hemorrhage and ensuring hemodynamic stability; maintaining spinal precautions; and providing oxygen therapy and fluid infusion (based on local protocols).

Nor does rapid assessment and treatment of a critically injured trauma patient mean that the paramedic should cut corners on the thoroughness of physical examination. Overlooking the entrance or exit wound that leads to an open pneumothorax and life-threatening tension pneumothorax is not going to be offset by getting to the trauma center a minute or two sooner. It's akin to speeding (over aggressively) to the scene of an accident but never arriving to help because you have a collision yourself.

In this case, the entrance and exit wound from the gunshot indicate potential injury to organs in the upper abdominal quadrants. Pain referred to the top of the shoulders indicates irritation to the diaphragm (blood in the area), which is innervated by C3–C5 through the phrenic nerve. Trauma to the spleen should be suspected with referred pain to the left shoulder, which is known as Kehr's sign. Both liver and spleen, which are located in the upper abdomen, are at risk for extensive bleeding, since they are very vascular organs. In abdominal injuries, a bullet that crosses the midline, as in this case, often causes more severe injury than one that remains on the same side.

A high index of suspicion for spinal injury must be maintained when dealing with gunshot wounds to the trunk. As such, it is appropriate to take spinal precautions, as was done in this case.

After a rapid trauma assessment, with appropriate intervention and a focused exam establishing a base line from which to measure, it's time to get moving. Detailed secondary surveys, along with additional patient history, and care of non life-threatening injuries can be addressed, if time allows, en route.

During transport the main concern is the stability of the patient, which means reassessment of ABCs and monitoring vital signs. Communication with the receiving hospital (trauma center) is essential to ensuring continuity of care, since all critical trauma patients will require aggressive emergency department management and almost all abdominal gunshot wounds will require surgery.

In the face of mass casualties and the stress of a highly charged atmosphere is not an easy task to stay cool under pressure and focus on the job at hand. terans with experience are the best equipped at remaining calm and thinking arly, however all EMTs can get through it if they rely on the most important s they have, that being their knowledge, training, and professionalism.

Knowledge and training are not hard to define, but just what does it mean a professional? Is a professional simply someone being paid to do a job such is distinguished from an amateur? Can a volunteer not then be able laim to being a professional? This case started out with reference to , a burned-out paramedic who, if his patient care is indeed suffering because of his attitude, has definitely crossed the line to unprofessionalism. A negative job outlook, subtle or not so subtle, unflattering comments toward patients, their relatives, or others (e.g., derogatory comments on treating alcoholics or the homeless) are all signs of burn-out and are inherently at odds with the caring and compassionate viewpoint that has brought us all to this field in the first place. This is separate from "gallows humor," which in this profession can be an appropriate stress relief under the right circumstances.

Burn-out is a progressive disease and comes when expectations are not met and when the daily accumulation of stress overwhelms coping mechanisms and support systems. Avoidance of burn-out comes when the idealism that exists with all who enter the EMS field is tempered with realism. Know what you're getting into. Professionalism is the armor that protects us along the way and its polish and shine is personal integrity.

Management has not cornered the market on professionalism. Management often defines it in terms of specific agendas. Worried about organizational image, quality assurance, lawsuits, and bottom lines, management creates policies, most often in a response to an issue or incident (not always proactively). Despite the good intentions behind tham, rules and regulations alone are not going to define someone's self-image of being a professional.

Believing that you are a professional means valuing yourself and your work. If you respect yourself you'll gain the respect of others. Being someone who can be relied on, someone who can be counted on to do the right thing, is all part of being a professional. Also, in order to do your best for others, be honest enough to admit you can improve and work hard to keep updated. The medical field is constantly evolving; don't be left behind. It is important to remember that the responsibility to avoid burn-out and maintain a professional approach rests with the individual. Acting like a professional has the side benefit of spilling over into our personal lives.

Personal integrity is not something taught in school. The streets with their unpredictability will often be a paradox to the classroom setting. Experiencing a tragic event or coping with a chaotic situation can lead to short tempers, short cuts in patient care, sloppy forms, and other adverse effects. It is important to keep in mind why we signed up in the first place. It certainly wasn't for the fabulous salary, the long hours of shift work, or the ongoing stress that comes with the job.

Avoiding burn-out means quite simply maintaining a professional approach under all circumstances. To be a respected EMS professional mean adopting a standard of ethical conduct that allows the EMT to be credible, to b educated, to instill confidence, and to demonstrate compassion. These are t signs and symptoms of a professional and they are more in evidence throu out the industry than we realize.

Follow-Up

Mr. Garvey was re-evaluated in the ER and concluded to have internal abdominal hemorrhage with hypovolemic shock. Blood was drawn for type and cross-match, and he was sent on to surgery. Hemorrhage was controlled with repair to the liver and a spleenectomy. Fortunately, no further damage was discovered. Mr. Garvey was able to make a full recovery and was discharged after a short stay, in time to be present for a memorial service in honor of his slain co-workers.

Apparently the gunman had recently been let go from the high tech company following an acrimonious dispute over ownership of newly created software. He had a family of three children and had recently separated from his wife. It was also revealed that he was suffering from a bipolar disorder.

Fact from Fiction

Kinetic energy is mostly dependant on velocity and as such, firearms can be classified as low, medium, or high velocity. Handguns are considered low-to-medium velocity at less than 2,000 ft/sec, whereas most rifles are considered high velocity and capable of causing greater damage. All firearms are potentially lethal depending on the area struck.

Factors that contribute to body tissue damage include: the size of the bullet, which relates to the caliber and internal diameter of the barrel (basically the bigger the missile the greater the path of destruction); ammunition characteristics such as deformity of the bullet such as hollow point and soft nose, which flatten out and mushroom (dum-dum) on impact, creating greater surface area involvement; bullets designed to tumble or yaw (wobble), which will impart a wider path of destruction; fragmentation, which will create multiple paths of damage; whether the bullet (usually a lead alloy) has a semi-jacket, a full or partial copper or steel coat, which expands to add greater surface damage; the distance or range from the target, since air resistance will decrease the speed of the bullet at the time of impact (at forty yards the velocity may be half the initial muzzle velocity).

One of the most influential factors in contributing to tissue damage, as noted, is the speed or velocity of the missile. Cavitation is the result of a bullet traveling through tissue at a high speed, where pressure waves or shock waves create a wake of destruction behind the bullet path. In low-velocity weapons this cavity may be temporary as the elasticity of the tissue returns it to original position. In this situation entry wounds may be not be readily apparent and a thorough examination is essential. With high velocity the cavity will be extensive, with the tissue not rebounding to its original shape.

The cavity created may be four to six times the size of the bullet's front surface area. Hunting rifles and assault weapons are classic in the creation of this wide permanent track along the missile's path.

Besides gathering information on the type of weapon and ballistics, much can be learned from a detailed description of the wound itself. Entry wounds are usually smaller than exit wounds. Two wounds may indicate an entrance and exit wound or two entrance wounds, since not all entrance wounds have exits. Close range shots may have darkened or burned edges, whereas most exit wounds have a stellate (starburst) pattern of jagged edges.

Answer Key & Rationale

1. d) Abdominal examination starts with a visual inspection. Gunshot wounds (unlike in the movies) are not always obvious and close visual assessment is important. Look for possible distention and gain a baseline from which to compare over time. Distention is indicative of severe internal bleeding since up to 1.5 liters of blood may accumulate before noticeable distention occurs. Palpate side to side, noting whether the abdomen is soft, tender, or rigid. Auscultation of bowel sounds requires a full minute to be accurate, and whether they are hyperactive or hypoactive is not clinically significant and only serves to delay definitive treatment.

2. a) The more dense the tissue, the greater the damage to that tissue. A bullet entering the body may change paths, particularly if it deflects off bone. Spinal injuries are always a concern for gunshot victims regardless of entry and exit wounds. Over 90 percent of abdominal gunshot wounds will require surgery and should be transported stat. Wearing a so-called bulletproof vest is no guarantee of being injury-free. Besides the armor-piercing capability of some military assault weapons, there can also be cardiac and other organ contusion without penetration.

3. d); **4.** c)   The peritoneal space (true abdomen) contains the liver, spleen, stomach, gallbladder, small and large intestines, and female reproductive organs. The retroperitoneal space (behind the true abdomen) contains the kidneys, ureters, pancreas, abdominal aorta, and inferior vena cava, as we as the posterior portion of the duodenum, ascending and descendi colon. It could be argued that the bladder is part of the true abdomen, he ever since the bladder is not in direct contact with the peritoneal cavity generally considered retroperitoneal. The distinction between the two ties is important, since occult bleeding into the retroperitoneal space likely to produce abdominal distention and can easily go unnoticed

5. a) In the presence of altered level of consciousness and/or spinal inj below the level of the abdomen, tenderness becomes a vague s and reveals little in the way of conclusive injury to the abdomen. Little is gained, while precious time is lost through auscultation and percussion of the abdomen on scene. Signs of intra-abdominal injury usually develop slowly, however if they do develop quickly it is because significant injury has occurred. Probing abdominal wounds with finger or any instrument is contraindicated and would only serve to cause further injury and potentiate sepsis.

6. d) Decreased perfusion resulting in systemic tissue hypoxia will usually occur when the systolic pressure drops below 90. Oxygen 12–15 l/m by non-rebreather mask and IV fluids normal saline or Ringer's lactate should be infusing at a rate to maintain the systolic above 90. In cases of gunshot wounds to the abdomen with significant internal bleeding, stabilization may require two large-bore IV lines running wide open and may be provided en route so as not to delay transport. (Check local protocols since controversy does exist over the efficacy of infusion therapy. An increase in blood pressure following infusion may serve to add to blood loss. Fluid infusion may also reactivate a bleed). When running IVs, monitor for pulmonary edema, a sign that circulatory overload is taking place. Fluid by mouth is always contraindicated since surgery is most probable.

7. e) Injuries to the stomach, pancreas, small intestine, and colon may not be readily apparent, or may easily be masked by other, more obvious injuries. Late developing complications can be very serious, including the possibility of death, if allowed to go undetected.

8. e) The diaphragm, liver, spleen, and stomach are all protected in part by the lower ribs and can all be injured by them if enough force is applied. The abdominal organs most commonly injured by rib fractures are the liver and spleen, which are extremely vascular, risking significant internal hemorrhage.

9. e) The peritoneal cavity is sterile and once contaminated can result is peritonitis (inflammation of the peritoneum), sepsis (massive infection), and endotoxic (septic) shock. Although the onset of septic shock is somewhat delayed, once it is established, it is just as life-threatening as hypovolemic shock.

. d) Shock with an unexplained etiology, or a level of shock greater than can be explained by other injuries, is the clearest indication of internal injury. Rigidity, guarding, and distension are not all that common and while external bruising raises the suspicion level, it is not itself indicative of intra-abdominal bleeding. Rebound tenderness (pain on release of palpation) is a sign more often associated with peritonitis. Fresh blood in the peritoneal cavity may not irritate the peritoneum and does not always ad to peritonitis. A high index of suspicion for intra-abdominal bleeding should be maintained, nonetheless, for external bruising, abdominal derness, rebound tenderness, as well as guarding and rigidity.

11. c) According to the American College of Surgeons, Class I hemorrhage involves blood loss of up to 15 percent of circulatory volume, or approximately 750 ml in an adult. Compensation usually maintains vital signs within a normal range. Class II is moderate blood loss of 15 to 30 percent or 750 ml to 1,500 ml. The patient in this stage becomes anxious and restless. Heart rate is tachycardic; while the blood pressure may be normal, the pulse pressure (difference between systolic and diastolic) will be narrowed. Class III indicates major blood loss between 30 and 40 percent (1500 ml to 2000 ml). The patient is not only anxious but is becoming confused. Blood pressure drops with systolic below 100, and both heart rate (>120) and respiratory rate (>30) are significantly elevated. Capillary refill is prolonged (>2 sec). Class IV hemorrhage is greater than 40 percent blood loss, and it is here that the pulse is often weak and thready if palpable at all. The blood pressure will be 90 systolic or less (diastolic not often captured), with the patient very weak and becoming unresponsive. The patient at this point is no longer compensating for blood loss, but is entering a state of decompensation with systemic tissue hypoxia and metabolic acidosis.

12. b) Normal saline (.9NaCl) and lactated Ringer's solutions are crystalloids that contain electrolytes. They are isotonic and are preferred over glucose, because they remain in the vascular system and are more effective in increasing blood volume. Plasma contains clotting factors without platelets or red blood cells and can be used in the field. In the hospital whole blood or packed red blood cells (most of the plasma removed) with saline may be given to replace blood loss when significant anemia accompanies hypovolemia.

GLOSSARY

abruptio placentae – the premature detachment of the placenta. Signs and symptoms include sudden third-trimester bleeding and pain.

acidotic – pertaining to excessive acidity of body fluids. This is due to an excessive loss of bicarbonate, as in renal disease, or an accumulation of acids, as in diabetic acidosis or renal failure.

adenosine triphosphate – an enzyme most common to muscle cells. The muscle's energy is stored in this compound.

algesia – the sense of pain.

allergen – a substance capable of producing hypersensitivity (allergy).

ambient – pertaining to the surrounding environment in which a person lives and works.

amniotic fluid – fluid that originates from several fetal sources such as fetal urine and the fetal respiratory tract. Also serves to protect and cushion the fetus.

anaerobic metabolism – metabolism occurring in the absence of oxygen.

anaphylactic – manifestation of a severe allergic reaction due to a great sensitivity to foreign protein or other material.

anastomosis – communication between two vessels by means of connected channels.

aneurysm – caused when localized, abnormal dilation of the wall of an artery or vein forms a sac, which results in weakness of the vessel.

anorexia – lack of or loss of appetite for food.

anuria – complete shutdown of urine output of a kidney.

aphasic – without the ability to speak.

apraxia – a voluntary movement disorder in which proper use of an object cannot be carried out, even though its uses can be described.

rteriosclerosis – condition pertaining to hardening, thickening, or loss of elasticity to the walls of arteries.

hralgia – joint pain.

es – accumulation and effusion of serous fluid in the abdominal cavity.

ptomatic – producing no or without symptoms.

ait – an unsteady, uncoordinated walk.

ataxic respiration – irregular breathing pattern with short, rapid breathing containing pauses lasting several seconds. Also known as Biot's respiration.

atelectasis – condition in which the lungs of an infant remain unexpanded at birth.

auscultate – to listen for sounds within the body, usually with a stethoscope as a diagnostic tool.

Babinski's reflex – dorsiflexion of the big toe upon stimulation of the sole of the foot.

battle sign – bruising over the mastoid process resulting from a fracture to the temporal bone.

bilirubin – an orange- or yellow-colored bile pigment derived from hemoglobin. An excess or bilirubin in cells and tissues causes jaundice.

Biot's respiration – an irregular breathing pattern with short, rapid breathing containing pauses of several seconds. Also known as ataxic respiration.

bradycardic – relating to a slow heart rate.

cerebral hypoxia – a reduction of the oxygen supply to the cerebrum.

Cheyne-Stokes respirations – atypical breathing pattern with a period of apnea lasting ten to sixty seconds followed by gradually increasing respirations.

cholecystitis – gallbladder inflammation.

cirrhosis – inflammation of parts or interspaces of an organ, particularly the liver.

coagulopathy – a blood coagulation disorder.

conduction – the act of transmitting certain forms of energy from one part to another.

congenital – existing at the time of birth.

conjugate – to be joined or paired.

consensual – a type of reflex caused by indirect stimulation of a receptor. Example: pupillary constriction of one eye when the other is stimulated by light.

contracture – permanent abnormal shortening of muscle tissue.

contrecoup – an injury occurring at a site opposite the site of impact.

convection – the transfer of heat by the movement of heated particles in or gases.

convulsion – violent jerking or a series of jerkings of the body.

coup – local damage that occurs at the site of impact.

crepitation – a dry, crackling sound or sensation. Often the result of the ends of fractured bones grating together.

decalcification – loss of calcium salts from a bone or tooth.

decerbrate posturing – abnormal extension response of the arms with extension of the legs. Caused by a rise in intracranial pressure.

decompensation – the inability of the heart to maintain adequate circulation.

decorticate posturing – abnormal flexor responses of one or both arms with extension of the legs. Caused by a rise in intracranial pressure.

dialysis – the process of removing toxic materials from the blood by passing it through a semi-permeable membrane.

diaphoresis – sweating profusely.

diplopia – double vision.

dorsalis – pertaining to a position nearer to the back of the body.

dysarthria – a disturbance in the ability to speak.

dyscrasia – a synonym for disease.

dysmetria – the inability to control the distance, power, and speed of a movement.

dysphagia – difficulty swallowing.

dyspnea – shortness of breath.

dysuria – difficult or painful urination.

eclampsia – condition occurring during pregnancy. Presents with convulsions and coma.

edema – an accumulation of fluid in intracellular spaces of the body causing swelling.

empathetic – being sensitive to another's feelings.

encephalopathy – pertaining to any brain disorder.

epilepsy – a chronic disorder characterized by paroxysmal brain dysfunction usually associated with some alteration of consciousness.

epinephrine – catecholamine secretion of the adrenal medulla.

esic – occurring outside of an organ.

palsies – paralysis of the facial muscles.

– the act of bending.

Fowler position – an upright sitting position obtained by raising the head of the bed about twenty to thirty inches.

fulminant – occurring suddenly with great intensity.

gangrene – death of tissue due to obstruction or loss of blood supply.

gestation – the length of time from conception to birth.

glomeruli – small structures in the body of the kidneys made up of capillary blood vessels in a cluster.

glucose – a sugar that is the most important carbohydrate in body metabolism.

glyconeogenesis – the formation of glycogen from noncarbohydrate sources such as protein or fat.

glycogenolysis – the conversion of glycogen into glucose in the body tissues.

glycosuria – the condition of having glucose in the urine.

hematoma – a mass of blood confined to a tissue, organ, or space. The most common cause is a break in a blood vessel.

hemophiliac – a person suffering from an inherited blood coagulation disorder.

hemianopia – blindness in half the field of vision in one or both eyes.

hemoptysis – referring to the splitting of blood or blood-stained sputum.

hepatitis – inflammation of the liver sometimes due to toxic agents, but usually due to viral infection.

hepatomegaly – liver enlargement.

homeostasis – the state of balance in the internal environment of the body.

hyaline membrane disease – a respiratory disease occurring in newborn infants characterized by dyspnea, cyanosis, expiratory grunt, rapid respirations, and limpness.

hypercapnia – excessive carbon dioxide in the blood.

hypercarotenemia – yellowing of the skin caused by an elevated level of carotene in the blood.

hypertension – high blood pressure.

hypertrophy – enlargement of part of all of an organ.

hypoadrenalism – referring to adrenal insufficiency.

hypoglycemia – a lower than normal amount of glucose in the blood.

hypopituitarism – the condition caused by the diminished secretion of pituitary hormones.

hypotension – low blood pressure.

hypothyroidism – decrease in thyroid activity.

hypovolemic shock – a condition resulting from a decrease in the volume of circulating body fluid, thus causing inadequate tissue perfusion.

hypoxia – reduced oxygen supply to a tissue.

hypoxic drive – the stimulus to breathe that is the result of low arterial oxygen pressure.

idiopathic – used to denote a disease of unknown origin.

inebriation – intoxication.

insidious – coming on gradually.

interstitial – relating to the inside of a vessel or organ.

intracellular – within a cell.

intracranial – within the skull.

ipsilateral – on or affecting the same side.

ischemia – temporary deficiency of local blood supply, caused by the obstruction of circulation to a part.

jaundice – a yellow or greenish pigmentation of the skin caused by high plasma bilirubin concentrations.

ketoacidosis – acidosis, as in diabetes or starvation, caused by enhanced production of ketone bodies. Fruity breathe odor, Kussmaul's respiration, nausea with vomiting, and a decreased level of consciousness are characteristics of this disorder.

kinematics – the science concerned with the body's movements.

Kussmaul's repirations – an abnormally deep, very rapid, sighing respiratory pattern.

lacrimation – the discharge of tears.

lateral decubitis – to lay on either the right or left side of the body.

lethargy – a lowered level of consciousness causing drowsiness and listlessness.

losomes – separate particles in the cell that are part of the intracellular digestive system.

se – a vague feeling of uneasiness or general discomfort.

a – the passage of dark stools stained with blood.

ic acidosis – a decreased pH and bicarbonate concentration in the fluids. Several causes include renal disease, diarrhea, impaired liver on, and severe dehydration.

miosis – the contraction of a pupil.

myalgia – pain of the muscles.

mydriasis – the dilation of a pupil.

necrosis – the death of areas of tissue or bone.

neural – pertaining to nerves or the nervous system.

neuroglycopenia – chronic hypoglycemia to a degree sufficient enough to cause brain dysfunction. This results in personality changes and intellectual deterioration.

neuropathy – any nerve disease.

noxious – harmful or dangerous.

nystagmus – constant and involuntary movement of the eyeball.

obtundation – a clouding of the consciousness.

oliguria – decrease in the amount of urine formation in relation to a person's fluid intake.

orthopneic position – upright position assumed when there is difficulty breathing when lying flat.

orthostatic – relating to an upright position.

osteoblast – a bone-forming cell.

osteoclast – a large multinuclear cell formed in the marrow of growing bones.

osteomyelitis – inflammation of bone due to infection.

osteoporosis – softening of bone, most often seen in the elderly.

osteopathy – any disease that affects the bones.

otorrhea – a discharge from the ears that can be from either inflammation or trauma.

palpation – to examine by feeling with the hands.

pancreatitis – inflammation of the pancreas associated with abdominal distension and tenderness with nausea and vomiting.

paresis – incomplete or slight paralysis.

parathesia – an abnormal sensation, such as burning, or tingling.

Parkinson's disease – a chronic nervous disorder that is characterized by a slow spreading tremor, muscular weakness, and rigidity.

pedal – pertaining to the feet.

peripheral – pertaining to a position away from the center of the body.

periorbital ecchymosis – bruising around both eyes caused by a basilar skull fracture. Also referred to as raccoon eyes.

peritoneal – concerning or pertaining to the peritoneum.

placenta previa – condition resulting from the placenta becoming implanted in the lower uterine segment. Characterized by bright red, painless bleeding with the absence of uterine contractions.

pneumotaxic – concerned with regulating the respiratory rate.

polydipsia – chronic excessive thirst.

polyhydramnios – an excess of fluid in the amniotic sac during pregnancy.

polyphagia – chronic excessive eating.

polyuria – excessive secretion of urine.

postictal – the period of time following a seizure.

prodromal – a symptom that can indicate the onset of a disease.

proteinuria – an excess of proteins in the urine.

proximal – nearest the point of origin.

ptosis – prolapse or sinking down of an organ.

rales – fine, bubbling sounds heard on auscultation of the lung.

respiratory acidosis – condition caused by the retention of carbon dioxide due to inadequate pulmonary vetilation.

respiratory alkilosis – condition caused by hyperventilation. Symptoms include lightheadedness and fainting.

retinopathy – any non-inflammatory disease of the retina.

rhinorrhea – a free discharge of nasal mucus usually thin in nature.

sclera – the tough, white, fibrous tissue that covers the eyeball. Also referred to as the white of the eye.

epsis – the presence of disease-causing organisms in the blood or tissues.

pticemia – systemic disease caused by the spread of pathogenic bacteria in the circulating blood. Sometimes referred to as blood poisoning.

1elae – used to refer to conditions that follow a disease.

olence – prolonged drowsiness.

tion – marked slowing of the flow of blood in the vessels.

stridor – harsh, high-pitched sound due to respiratory obstruction.

stupor – the condition of a lower level of consciousness.

surfactant – any agent that lowers surface tension.

syncope – fainting.

tachycardic – relating to a rapid heart rate.

tachypnea – rapid breathing.

thermoregulation – temperature control.

tinnitus – the condition of hearing noises in the ear such as ringing, buzzing, or roaring.

toxemia – the condition resulting from the circualtion of toxins by the blood-stream.

transient monocular blindness – short-lived blindness in one eye.

tremulousness – trembling.

trendelenburg – position where the bed is raised so the feet and pelvis are higher than the head.

uremia – the excess of urea in the blood.

vasoconstriction – narrowing of blood vessels.

vasodilation – the dilation or widening of the lumen of blood vessels.

vasodilator – any substance that causes dilation of the blood vessels.

venostasis – the slowing of venous outflow in a body part.